Praise for *The Elderberry Book*

As a long-time cultivator of elderberry, for not only its beauty
as part of my farm landscape but also for making pancake syrup and
tinctures, I had a hunch there was plenty I didn't know. John Moody
has given me a new set of eyes, plus the tools, recipes, and step-by-
step how-to for utilizing every part of my beloved elder.

MARYJANE BUTTERS Idaho farmer, author, and editor of *MaryJanesFarm*
magazine, now in its 19th year, and author, *Wild Bread*

John Moody remains one of the important voices in the modern
homesteading and regenerative agriculture movements. With a style that
blends practical knowledge with front porch philosophy, in *The Elderberry
Book* you'll learn all the necessary information on how to use one of
my favorite plants for food and forage, drink and medicine.

SCOTT MANN host, The Permaculture Podcast

The elderberry is a great plant to fall in love with;
this book is its love letter to everybody.

SAMUEL THAYER author, *Nature's Garden,
The Forager's Harvest*, and *Incredible Wild Edibles*

John Moody has done an excellent job in profiling the many aspects of the lore, cultivation and use of this amazing specialty fruit in an easy-to-understand but professional manner. Always a plant of the people, elderberry has been used for healing since earliest times in a diversity of human practices and preferences. As a practical guide for home or small farm production, this book a great place to start.

CHRIS PATTON Founder and President of
the Midwest Elderberry Cooperative

John dives into elderberries with the same enthusiasm he brings to the homesteading lifestyle. From plant to product, *The Elderberry Book* has you covered. It was fun and entertaining to learn about new aspects of an old herbal friend, the elderberry.

LAURIE NEVERMAN founder, Common Sense
Home, blogger at commonsensehome.com

the
elderberry
book

forage • cultivate • prepare • preserve

John Moody

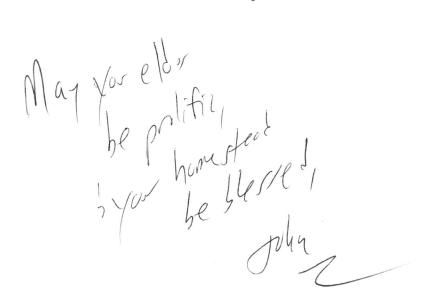

May you elder
be prolific,
& your homestead
be blessed,

John

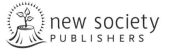

new society
PUBLISHERS

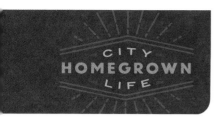

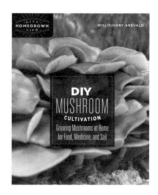

Y OU'D LIKE TO be self-sufficient, but the space you have available is tighter than your budget. If this sounds familiar, the **Homegrown City Life Series** was created just for you! Our authors bring country living to the city with big ideas for small spaces. Topics include cheesemaking, fermenting, gardening, composting and, more—everything you need to create your own homegrown city life!

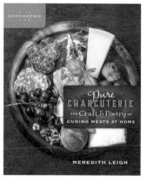

- **The Food Lover's Garden:** *Growing, Cooking and Eating Well* by Jenni Blackmore

- **The Art of Plant-Based Cheesemaking,** revised & updated 2nd edition: *How to Craft Real, Cultured, Non-Dairy Cheese* by Karen McAthy

- **Worms at Work:** *Harnessing the Awesome power of Worms with Vermiculture and Vermicomposting* by Crystal Stevens

- **Pure Charcuterie:** *The Craft and Poetry of Curing Meats at Home* by Meredith Leigh

- **DIY Kombucha:** *Sparkling Homebrews Made Easy* by Andrea Potter

- **DIY Mushroom Cultivation:** *Growing Mushrooms at Home for Food, Medicine, and Soil* by Willoughby Arevalo

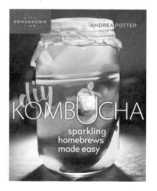

FORTHCOMING

- **DIY Autoflowering Cannabis** by Jeff Lowenfells

- **Your Indoor Herb Garden** by DJ Herda

- **DIY Sourdough** by John and Jessica Moody

#homegrowncitylife

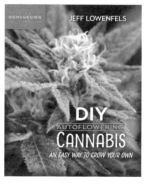

Cover design by Diane McIntosh.
Cover Image © iStock.

Printed in Canada. Second printing July 2020.

Inquiries regarding requests to reprint all or part of *The Elderberry Book* should be addressed to New Society Publishers at the address below. To order directly from the publishers, please call toll-free (North America) 1-800-567-6772, or order online at www.newsociety.com

Any other inquiries can be directed by mail to:
New Society Publishers
P.O. Box 189, Gabriola Island, BC V0R 1X0, Canada
(250) 247-9737

LIBRARY AND ARCHIVES CANADA CATALOGUING IN PUBLICATION

Title: The elderberry book : forage, cultivate, prepare, preserve / John Moody.
Names: Moody, John (Homesteader), author.
Description: Includes bibliographical references and index.

Identifiers: Canadiana (print) 20190128062 | Canadiana (ebook) 20190128070 |
    ISBN 9780865719194 (softcover) | ISBN 9781550927122 (PDF) |
    ISBN 9781771423083 (EPUB)

Subjects: LCSH: Elders (Plants)

Classification: LCC QK495.A178 M66 2019 | DDC 583/.987—dc23

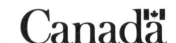

Funded by the Government of Canada   Financé par le gouvernement du Canada

New Society Publishers' mission is to publish books that contribute in fundamental ways to building an ecologically sustainable and just society, and to do so with the least possible impact on the environment, in a manner that models this vision.

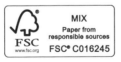

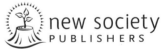

"Lady Ellhorn, give me of thy wood,
And I will give thee of mine,
When I become a tree."

"And thus the king and his knights
were turned to stone and the witch
turned herself into an elder tree."

ARTHUR EVANS *Folklore*, 1865

Contents

Acknowledgments

MY MANY THANKS to all those who perused the manuscript, helped hunt down some of the harder to find historical information, and otherwise supported this effort. I hope in years to come we see an elderberry bush on every corner, and better health to our homes, homesteads, and home countries because of it.

For those who lack classical libraries, you can access many ancient herbal and medicinal texts through services such as Perseus at Tufts University and the Loeb Classical Library. My thanks to Dr. Peter Gentry and Dr. John Meade for their assistance.

Another organization that also preserves and makes available historical documents of interest is Archive.org. Without their work, this book would be bereft of dozens of photos, quotes, and research that showcases the history, usefulness, and ubiquity of the elder over the past four centuries.

Another of note is the Missouri Botanical Garden, which preserves a great wealth of information and imagery of our world's amazing flora. Thank you Catherine Martin for your help in acquiring images that have enriched this publication and for work that enriches our world. Also, thanks to Natalie Carmolli at Proven Winners, who provided images of some unique ornamental elder varieties; it is also a place where you can acquire such unique elder cultivars.

To Nick, John, Alan, and many others who proofed sections of or the entire book, or helped me in so many other ways, my deepest thanks. To the many farmers and friends who helped me with pictures I couldn't get because of the time of year I wrote the book— thank you! If you are looking to purchase an elder, please consider supporting these farmers. To Chris Patton of the Midwest Elderberry Cooperative, my appreciation for reviewing some of the technical info in the book, offering suggestions, and for all I have learned from your organization's research and work.

To my wife and kids, thank you for putting up with me making a mess of the house and kitchen repeatedly, and running out and interrupting life and school every time I found some new nugget of elder lore that I found of interest. To all my friends at New Society, especially Ingrid for patiently chasing me around fairs for a few years, thank you for two wonderful book projects.

To you the reader, my gratitude for choosing this book among the ocean available. I poured a good bit of my life and soul into this book, and I hope that it enriches your life, soul, and land for many years to come.

Introduction

MANY YEARS AGO, after we had settled onto our first homestead, a friend came out to visit. As Ben and I walked around the property, he bent down here, or reached there, collecting what seemed to me to be nothing but weeds or bark or other scraps of plants and vegetation. Or he would point at some mass of tangled green growing things, mentioning a number of names that made no sense to me at the time, rattling off different ways they could be used as food or medicine.

Ben was a forager, someone intimately familiar with the benefits of the abundant plant life all around us, something that most of us—including our family at the time—completely missed. Queen Anne's Lace and plantain. Wood sorrell and wild hickory (pig nut). Elderberry and acorns. Some are food. Some are medicine. Many are both.

If you are reading this book, then my hunch is you either already are into or are interested in learning more about such things—foraging, food as medicine, perennial plants with a rich culinary, craft, and medicinal history; creating a more sufficient farm or homestead, and much more. So, I want to start with a suggestion. Once you finish learning about elderberry, don't stop! Elderberry is just one, albeit an exceptional one, of so many plants surrounding us that have innumerable benefits. Start with elderberry, but continue to learn, plant, forage, enrich, and explore long after.

The book follows a simple structure. It will start with just a brief survey of our long relationship with elder. We will cross time, cultures, and continents. Then, we will briefly look at elder's anatomy and terminology so that later in the book and out in the fields and forests, you better understand how to find and identify it. Next, we will talk about how to tend elderberry, from different ways to plant and propagate it to the most common diseases and pests that may afflict it. This naturally leads into a discussion on harvesting elderberries—both by foraging for them or from your own plantings. Since elderberries occur in abundance, knowing how to preserve the harvest comes immediately after. Last, we will look at the myriad ways elderberry can be used, both culinary and craft. By the end, I hope you will have a deeper appreciation for one of God's great gifts, the elder tree.

There was a great deal I couldn't fit into this introductory book, so if you want to learn more or connect, visit www.theelderberrybook.com

History

IN A HUMBLE 17th-century western European village, a grandma makes elderberry tea for her sick grandson. In a Mediterranean house in the 10th century, a man uncorks last year's elderberry wine, now ready to enjoy over dinner with friends. In a Roman town in 223 AD, a physician makes a paste of elderberry leaves and other herbs to apply to an unknown skin infection on his patient. On the Great Plains of America, an Indian cuts wood from a bush to fashion into a new flute for his son, while in Greece a young lady plays the *sambuke*, a wooden stringed instrument.

What do these people, diverse through time and geography, have in common? A native plant known by many, many names—Arbre de Judas, Baccae, Baies de Sureau, Black-Berried Alder, Black Elder, Boor Tree, Bountry, Elder, Common Elder, Ellanwood, Ellhorn, European Alder, Fruit de Sureau, Grand Sureau, Hautbois, Holunderbeeren, Sabugeuiro-negro, Sambequier, Sambu, Sambuc, Sambuci, Sambucus, Sambucus nigra, Sambugo, Sauco, Saúco Europeo, Schwarzer Holunder, Seuillet, Seuillon, Sureau, Sureau Européen, Sureau Noir, Sus, Suseau, Sussier. To us, it is known as the elder or elderberry.

If the dog is humanity's best friend, then the elderberry may be its best plant friend, for this plant has been a part of our lives for many thousands of years. Let's look at our long relationship with the elder.

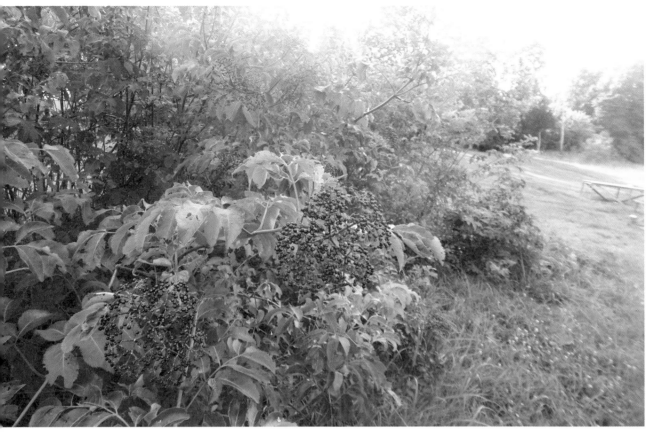

▲ The elder.

ANCIENT ELDERBERRY

Few plants have received the amount of attention across peoples and places like elder. Also, few plants have been with us as long—archaeological evidence has found elder seeds in sites over 9,000 years old. It makes sense. Few plants provide one-stop shopping like the elder. It is fruit, medicine, and craft, all in one fast-growing and resilient plant.

Since written sources are somewhat scarce for earlier periods, we will start with where elder, especially as used and understood today, begins: the Greek and Roman cultures. The founders of modern botany, pharmacology, herbology, and medicine all discuss, often at length, the elder.

Hippocrates, often called the "Father of Medicine," has many comments about making use of the elder's root, leaves, and juice. The leaves occur far more often than any other part.

> Every third day, let him bathe, if it helps; if not let him be anointed; also let him take walks, if he is able, determining their distance in accordance with his food. Boil leaves of the elder tree and of the fleabane that is always tender, and give these to the patient to drink.[1]

19. If the brain suffers from bile, a mild fever is present, chills, and pain through the whole head, especially in the temples, bregma, and the sockets of the eyes. The eyebrows seem to overhang, pain sometimes migrates to the ears, bile runs out through the nostrils, and the patient sees unclearly. In most patients, pain occupies one half of the head, but it can also arise in the whole head.

When the case is such, apply cold compresses to the patient's head, and, when the pain and flux cease, instill celery juice into his nostrils. Let him avoid bathing, as long as the pain is present, take as gruel thin millet to which a little honey has been added, and drink water. If nothing passes off below, have him eat cabbage, and drink the juice as gruel; if not that, then the juice of elder leaves in the same way. When you think it is the right moment, give foods of the most laxative kind.[2]

Treat persons suffering from wounds by having them abstain from food, by administering an enema or giving a medication to evacuate the contents downwards from their cavity, and by having them drink water and vinegar, and take watery gruel. If the wound is inflamed, cool it with plasters; let the plasters be made from beets boiled in water, or celery, or olive leaves, or fig leaves, or leaves of elder or bramble, or sweet pomegranate; apply these boiled.[3]

HIPPOCRATES

Galen, one of the most prolific writers in all of ancient history (roughly half of all the literature we have from ancient Greece is attributed to him!), was a Greek physician and surgeon from 129 to 200 AD. He quoted Hippocrates often, and also added to some of the then commonly accepted uses of elder in medicine.

107 Danewort/Dwarf Elder and Elder

Danewort and elder may differ in size but they are similar in their leaves, flower, and seed, and they have almost the same properties. The root of danewort is especially good for clearing up and purging dropsy, and its leaves when cooked and eaten purge the bowels.[4]

Theophrastus, the famous Greek botanist, mentions elder a number of times, noting that it grew "chiefly by water," something we discuss later when it comes to cultivating the plant. He also made many medicinal observations, though none about elderberry proper, noting that the best plant juices were collected during summer, whereas the best roots for medicinal use came in the spring and fall.

Again some are without knots, as the stems of elder, others have knots, as those of fir and silver-fir … Again there are differences in the "core": in the first place according as plants have any or have none, as some say is the case with elder among other things; and in the second place there are differences between those which have it, since in different plants it is respectively fleshy, woody, or membranous; fleshy, as in vine fig apple pomegranate elder ferula; woody, as in Aleppo pine silver-fir fir; in the last-named especially so, because it is resinous.[5]

Dioscorides, a Greek doctor and pharmacologist who lived from around 40 to 90 BC, is the author of *De Materia Medica*, or *On Medical Material*. This illustrated five-volume book series was hand copied in Latin, Greek, and Arabic, and circulated all the way into

THAT PLANT OF GOD THAT HEALS ALL THINGS?
A number of quotes are attributed to Hippocrates regarding elder. After extensive searching, I was unable to confirm two in particular, "the plant of God that heals everything it touches" and the "medicine chest of the people." I used a number of tools to try and confirm these quotes, including getting assistance from three different professors with specialties in the classics and ancient Near Eastern history, and still came up empty. This doesn't mean that these two quotes are spurious, just that they may not belong to Hippocrates but some other person and ended up attributed to him, or that they do belong to him, but the original texts were lost and only secondhand sources remain for these attributions. Given that, for Galen and many Greek authors, we sometimes have a third or less of their total writings intact, this is quite possible. If anyone has access to any first or secondhand sources that use these quotes, please contact me.

the Middle Ages as the standard text covering around 600 plants and over 1,000 medicines made from them. Elderberry is listed in Book Four along with over half a dozen uses, from treating skin ailments to dropsy. Every part of the plant is discussed, from root to leaf:

> This has the same properties and uses as that above—drying, expelling water, yet bad for the stomach. The leaves (boiled as vegetables) purge phlegm and bile, and the stalks (boiled as a vegetable) do the same. The roots (boiled with wine and given with meat) are good for dropsy. A decoction (taken as a drink) helps those bitten by vipers. Boiled with water for bathing it softens the womb and opens the vagina, and sets to rights any disorders around it. A decoction of the fruit (taken as a drink with wine) does the same things, and rubbed on it darkens the hair. The new tender leaves (smeared on with polenta) lessen inflammation, and smeared on, they are good for burns and dog bites. Smeared on with bull or goat grease they heal hollow ulcers, and help gout. It is also called heliosacte, sylvestris sambucus, or euboica; the Romans call it ebulus, the Gauls, ducone, and the Dacians, olma.[6]

Pliny the Elder, who lived from around 23 to 79 AD, was a noted Roman writer and scholar. His *On the Materials of Medicine* devotes an entire chapter to the elder:

Chapter 35. The Elder, Fifteen Remedies

> A decoction of the leaves, seed, or root of either kind, taken in doses of two cyathi, in old wine, though bad for the upper regions of the stomach, carries off all aqueous humours by stool. This decoction is very cooling too for inflammations, those attendant upon recent burns in particular. A poultice is made also of the more tender leaves, mixed with polenta, for bites inflicted by dogs. The juice of the elder, used as a fomentation, reduces abscesses of the brain, and more particularly of the membrane which envelopes that organ. The berries, which have not so powerful an action as the other parts

of the tree, stain the hair. Taken in doses of one acetabulum, in drink, they are diuretic. The softer leaves are eaten with oil and salt, to carry off pituitous and bilious secretions. The smaller kind is for all these purposes the more efficacious of the two. A decoction of the root in wine, taken in doses of two cyathi, brings away the water in dropsy, and acts emolliently upon the uterus: the same effects are produced also by a sitting-bath made of a decoction of the leaves. The tender shoots of the cultivated kind, boiled in a sauce-pan and eaten as food, have a purgative effect: the leaves taken in wine, neutralize the venom of serpents. An application of the young shoots, mixed with he-goat suet, is remarkably good for gout; and if they are macerated in water, the infusion will destroy fleas. If a decoction of the leaves is sprinkled about a place, it will extermi-nate flies. "Boa" is the name given to a malady which appears in the form of red pimples upon the body; for its cure the patient is scourged with a branch of elder. The inner bark, pounded and taken with white wine, relaxes the bowels.[7]

Also note, while the literature of the time primarily concerns itself with elder as medicine, its many other uses were well known and appreciated. For instance, even Pliny appears to have commented on elderberry's use for whistles and popguns, one that endured deep into American history. Also, he is one of the earliest to record elderberry's use as a hair dye.[8] These early works and studies on elderberry set the stage for most of the rest of its history and use—direct quotations and echoes of their work will appear in almost all writings on elder-berry to this day.

The modern names for the tree also have Greco-Roman roots. Elder comes from *aeld* or *ellarn*, a word that meant "to kindle or fire." Its long hollow stems are excellent for blowing air into a fire from a distance. Greek mythology shows that it may be one of the earliest uses of the plant. Prometheus, who gave the gift of fire to humanity, is said to have carried his gift in a hollowed-out branch, a branch that was perhaps fashioned from the elder.

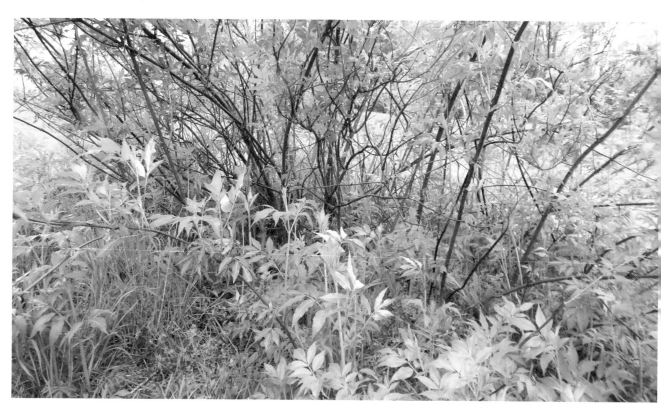

▲ The elder's habit of growing twisted and tangled led to its association with ill luck and misfortune.

EUROPEAN ELDERBERRY

While Greco-Roman culture and influence waxed and waned, the centrality of elderberry as a useful medicine has endured right up until modern times. The peasant's medicine chest had real staying power. At the same time, elderberry was deeply entwined in the superstitions and religious scruples of the different countries where it grew.

While esteemed for its healing properties, elder was also viewed with skepticism and fear. It didn't help that Judas Iscariot was said to have hanged himself from an elder tree, a story some say was invented to discourage tree worship, especially of the elder. The old rhyme, "Bour tree, bour tree, crooked, wrong, / Never straight and never strong, Never bush and never tree, / Since our Lord was nailed on thee," is just one of many examples of how elder became entwined with negative associations.[9]

Such myths expanded over time in Europe, where the wood of the elder became associated with witches, ill luck, and bad omens in many countries. In Shakespeare's play *Cymbeline*, elderberry appears as a symbol of sadness and grief.[10] Yet, Shakespeare also shows the great esteem elderberry was held in by the people when one of his characters compares it to the greatest healers of antiquity: "What says my Aesculapius? my Galen? my heart of Elder?" (*Merry Wives of Windsor*, Act II, Sc. 3).

It is here, in European history, that we find what is most likely the earliest recorded mention of the use of elderberry juice to increase resistance to illness, from German scholar Conrad von Megenberg (1309–1374).

Many books were written about elder's properties across Europe. Their titles match the great esteem the plant had received for the past 1,000 years. One of the most noteworthy is *The Anatomy of the Elder Cutting Out of It Plain, Approved, and Specific Remedies for Most and Chiefest Maladies: Confirmed and Cleared by Reason, Experience, and History* by Martin Blochwich. Written in 1644, it is probably the earliest work devoted solely to elder's medical use. In it, he draws heavily on the writings of those mentioned above but adds a great deal more to the already extensive discussion of elderberry—the book tallies over 250 pages!

> If the medicinal properties of its leaves, bark and berries were fully known, I cannot tell what our countryman could ail for which he might not fetch a remedy from every hedge, either for sickness, or wounds.[11]
>
> **JOHN EVELYN**

Also, elder wasn't just for the learned. It was truly "the medicine chest of the country people"—an appellation we can first credit to 16th-century doctor, Michael Ettmeuller.[12]

It is of no surprise that, alongside technical treatises on the plant, we find fairy tales and other fanciful stories, folk remedies, traditional recipes, and dozens of other uses. The 1852 *Flora Homoeopathica* recounts, "It was the chief ingredient in Lady Mary Douglas's specific; and Elder-flower water and Elder-flower ointment were in every domestic medicine case; the North American Indians make an eye-water from the young leaves of the Elder."[13]

On the fairy-tale side, one of the most memorable, and accessible, is that of "The Elder-Tree Mother" by Hans Christian Andersen. While mainly known for tales such as "The Emperor's New Clothes," "The Little Mermaid," and "The Ugly Duckling," he also included one about the elder:

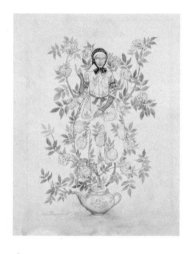

In the Midst of the Tree Sat a Kindly Old Woman, by Arthur Rackham. England, 1939
From *The Little Elder Tree Mother*

And the little boy looked toward the teapot. He saw the lid slowly raise itself and fresh white elder flowers come forth from it. They shot long branches even out of the spout and spread them abroad in all directions, and they grew bigger and bigger until there was the most glorious elderbush—really a big tree! The branches even stretched to the little boy's bed and thrust the curtains aside—how fragrant its blossoms were! And right in the middle of the tree there sat a sweet-looking old woman in a very strange dress. It was green, as green as the leaves of the elder tree, and it was trimmed with big white elder blossoms; at first one couldn't tell if this dress was cloth or the living green and flowers of the tree.

"What is this woman's name?" asked the little boy.

"Well, the Romans and the Greeks," said the old man, "used to call her a 'Dryad,' but we don't understand that word. Out in New Town, where the sailors live, they have a better name for her. There she is called 'Elder Tree Mother,' and you must pay attention to her; listen to her, and look at that glorious elder tree![14]

HANS CHRISTIAN ANDERSEN *"The Little Elder Tree Mother"*

The association of elder with magic spanned countries and cultures in Europe. Lady Northcote, who in 1903 wrote *The Book of Herbs*, collected dozens of pieces of lore around the elder. Summing up many hundreds of years of European history, she writes, "Every inch of the Elder-tree is connected with magic."[15]

Some of these myths and stories are quite serious, while others, rather humorous. For instance, one recounts how elder was the perfect wood for making stakes to use against vampires—a serious fear in parts of Europe for some two hundred years. Another, drawing on the legend that vampires must compulsively count all things—an idea that I was exposed to as a child by the television show *Sesame Street*—said to leave the berries on your windowsill. A vampire seeking to enter your residence would be kept preoccupied until morning tallying the berries before they could enter. Two forms of defense from a single plant!

Nicholas Culpeper, a doctor in England in the 1600s, also points to how well established the elder was in common knowledge. His work, along with that of Sauer, were the go-to home remedy books for over a hundred years in parts of Europe and the United States.

Culpeper notes that *"Elder flowers*, help dropsies, cleanse the blood, clear the skin, open stoppings of the liver and spleen, and diseases arising therefrom."

Rob Baccarum Sambuci or Rob of Elder Berries

College.] Take of the juice of Elder Berries, and make it thick with the help of a gentle fire, either by itself, or a quarter of its weight in sugar being added.

Culpeper.] Both Rob of Elder Berries, and Dwarf-Elder, are excellent for such whose bodies are inclining to dropsies, neither let them neglect nor despise it. They may take the quantity of a nutmeg each morning, it will gently purge the watery humour.[17]

This rob—a rob is a thick, heavily reduced juice and sweetener—was sometimes added to warm water or tea and taken for coughs, colds, and flu. It is in some ways the predecessor to our modern elderberry syrups.

I hold it needless to write any description of this, since every boy that plays with a pop-gun will not mistake another tree instead of Elder.[16]

NICHOLAS CULPEPER

Culpeper also notes elder's effectiveness for treating toothache:

8. For the Tooth-Ache

Take the inner rind of an Elder-tree, and bruise it, and put thereto a little Pepper, and make it into balls, and hold them between the teeth that ache.

Elder wasn't just a home remedy, though. Numerous products were made using elder and elderberry, from non-alcoholic beverage to body care.

John Parkinson (1567–1650) was apothecary to James I and a founding member of the Worshipful Society of Apothecaries. He is celebrated for his two monumental works, the first *Paradisi in Sole Paradisus Terrestris* in 1629 (a gardening book), but the second was his *Theatrum Botanicum* of 1644, one of the largest herbals ever produced. A portion of this book was dedicated entirely to the virtues of the elder tree, wherein the author sings its praises in no less than 230 pages. That portion of the book became so popular that a booklet of that section was published in several editions in both English and Latin. Every single part of the plant was mentioned as medicinally useful. Its medicinal powers were deemed effective for treating quinsy (peritonsillar abscesses), sore throats, and strangulation. The elderberries were also used for practically any ailment, "from toothache to the plague." It seems like a whole apothecary could be stocked solely from the many preparations that could be made from its various parts. The list is quite exhaustive—syrup, tincture, mixture, oil, ointment, concoction, liniment, extract, salt, conserve, vinegar, oxymel, sugar, decoction, bath, cataplasm, and powder made from one, several, or all parts of the plant.[18]

"The people's medicine chest" was still going strong in the early 1800s. *The American Frugal Housewife*, written by Lydia Child in 1835, speaks of the many uses of elder, not just as drink or medicine but also as insect repellent and plant protection. Echoing earlier works, she says of the elder: "Every part of it serves some useful purpose—the wood, pith, bark, leaves, buds, flowers, and fruit."[19]

In 1895, *The Cottage Physician: Best Known Methods of Treatment in All Diseases, Accidents and Emergencies of the Home,* by Dr. Thomas Faulkner and Dr. John H. Carmichael, said of elderberry that it was a "rather laxative and also act[s] upon the skin. They are often used in treating rheumatism, gout, scrofula and habitual constipation." The elder—mainly as flower—is mentioned around a dozen times, for such disparate ailments as earaches, eye issues, constipation, bone ulcers, measles, and dropsy.[20]

In its reference section, instructions include how to make a diaphoretic decoction (a herbal or medicine that induces sweating) using 1 to 2 tablespoons of elderflowers steeped in water. Decoctions are similar to teas, and the manual even mentions the addition of honey in some situations. "From one to four tablespoons of the expressed juice of the inner bark of the elder, taken every four hours, till it operates freely, is of great service."[21]

The culinary value of elderberry was not lost as time progressed, either. It was especially valued in winemaking, with many recipes for both the flowers and berries continually circulated throughout Europe and America for hundreds of years.

438. To Make Elder-Flower Wine

Take three or four handfuls of dry'd elder-flowers, and ten gallons of spring water, boil the water, and pour in scalding hot upon the flowers, the next day put to every gallon of water five pounds of Malaga raisins, the stalks being first pick'd off, but not wash'd, chop them grosly with a chopping knife, then put them into your boiled water, stir the water, raisins and flowers well together, and do so twice a day for twelve days, then press out the juice clear as long

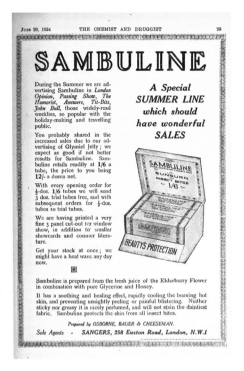

THE CHEMIST AND DRUGGIST, 1924.
ARCHIVE.ORG

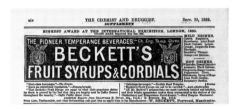

THE CHEMIST AND DRUGGIST, 1889.
ARCHIVE.ORG

as you can get any liquor; put it into a barrel fit for it, stop it up two or three days till it works, and in a few days stop it up close, and let it stand two or three months, then bottle it.[22]

Indeed, it is hard to find any book about winemaking that didn't include the elder! Most older cookbooks and winemaking guides contained at a minimum two, with many having four or more recipes that include elderflowers or berries. But wine alone wasn't on the menu. Works spanning the 1400s and onward include directions for elderberry brandy, mead, and cordials, along with jams and jellies. A few even include rather unique dishes, such as elderberry soup.

I would be remiss to not mention my favorite reference to elderberry in more recent European literature: Monty Python's "Your mother was a hamster, and your father smells of elderberry." Tragedy, comedy, poetry, even deft insult is all a part of elder's rich history and lore.

NATIVE AMERICAN AND AMERICAN ELDERBERRY

Elderberry's history in North America is not as well known but no less rich than in Europe. The Native Americans made use of elderberry far back into their histories. Indeed, elderberry was present at the beginning of history:

The Birth of Wek'-Wek and the Creation of Man

Its branches, as they swayed in the wind, made a sweet musical sound. The tree sang; it sang all the time, day and night, and the song was good to hear. Wik'-wek looked and listened and wished he could have the tree. Near by he saw two Hol-luk'-ki or Star-people, and as he looked he perceived that they were the Hul-luk mi-yum'-ko— the great and beautiful women-chiefs of the Star-people. One was the Morning Star, the other Pleiades Os-so-so'-li. They were watching and working close by the elderberry tree. Wek'-wek liked the music and asked the Star-women about it. They told him that the tree whistled songs that kept them awake all day and all night so

they could work all the time and never grow sleepy. They had the
rattlesnakes to keep the birds from carrying off the elderberries.[23]

To the various native tribes, the elderberry was associated with
trustworthiness and honesty:

> On this journey some of the personal delegation to communicate
> with Hiawatha used for a pledge small shoots from the elderberry
> bush which were cut into short pieces, and from which the pith was
> removed, and those little cylinders strung on small cords of sinew.
> Likewise, the tradition continues, the quills of large feathers, cut
> and strung on cords, were also used as tokens, pledges, or vouches
> for the good faith of the messenger or speaker.[24]

Elder's use in the Americas is as old or older than in European and
Mediterranean peoples—archeologists have recovered its seeds dat-
ing between 1000 to 1300 BC at various Native American sites. One
of the world's earliest on-the-go snack bars—pemmican, a mixture of
bison or beef fat and dried, finely pounded meat—would sometimes
include elderberries. Most other uses found in America mirror those
of Europe: musical instruments and other hand tools, beverages of
many kinds, and even clusters of flowers battered and fried developed among the Native Americans, just as among the Greco-Roman
cultures. The medicinal uses also closely mirrored those practiced on
the other side of the world—treatment for fevers, purgatives, the bark
for wounds, sores, and other skin ailments; every part of the plant
was prized medicine.[25]

The colonists brought some European cultivars over, but also
quickly learned to make use of the native elder found across the continent. It is hard to find a culinary or medicinal text from the first 150
years of US history that doesn't mention elder. During the Civil War,
along with many other native plants, the elder was relied on heavily
by both Union and Confederates. As the war carried on, medicines
became scarce, especially in the South, so soldiers and physicians

began to fall back on herbal lore and whatever plants the landscape provided:

> I enumerate a few more medicinal uses that were made of some of the products of our Southern fields and forests by our physicians and housewives… A decoction made by pouring boiling water over the leaves, flowers or berries of the elder bush was used as a wash for wounds to prevent injuries from flies.[26]

Because of its color and flavor, elderberry was sometimes also used as an adulterate (not necessarily in the modern negative sense of the word) in wines and other beverages, so well-trained barkeepers, buyers, and butlers were taught how to detect its presence.[27]

MORE THAN JUST FOOD OR MEDICINE

While elderberry has a long, rich, and deep history of culinary and medicinal use, the plant was prized for many other purposes as well. The word *elder* is thought to come from or be related to the old word *aeld*, meaning "fire or wind." Some of the earliest recorded uses are as bellows for blowing air into a fire along with musical instruments. Indeed, the Greek and Latin root for elder, *sambu,* appears to have originally referred to a flute-like instrument made from elder wood.

Elderberry was often used as a dye for fabrics but wasn't limited solely to paints and clothing. It also works as a food dye, such as for coloring things like Easter eggs or cake frosting. People also used elderberry as a hair dye, for complexion and skin, and as makeup.[29] If you deal with elderberry on a regular basis, you will quickly realize that, even if it doesn't heal everything it touches, it will stain it!

Because of its beauty and growth habit, for at least 2,000 years, people have used elderberry in landscaping and homestead design; similar to flutes and popguns, it is mentioned all the way back in Greco-Roman times. It is one of the earliest plants used by people to create what are now sometimes called "living fences." In the *Systematic Agriculture: The Mystery of Husbandry Discovered,* written by

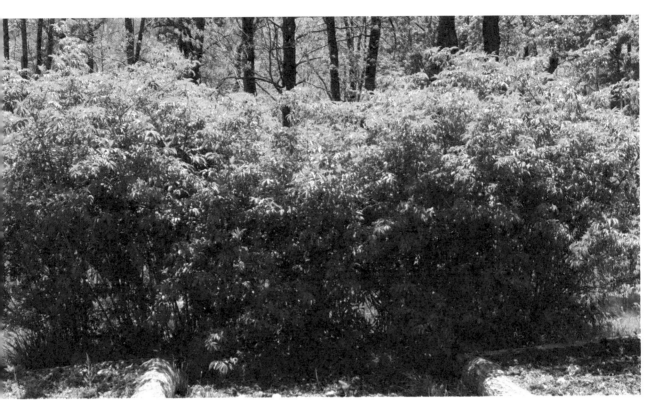

▲ Elder create wonderful screens and hedges. CHERIE MCDIFFETT, RUSTIC
ACRES FARM

John Worlidge around 1675, the elder is included with "trees necessary and proper for fencing and enclosing of Lands":

> A considerable Fence may be made of Elder, set of reasonable hasty
> Truncheons, like the Willow and may be laid with great curiosity:
> this makes a speedy shelter for a garden from Winds, Beasts and
> such like injuries, rather than from rude minchers.[30]

Because of the plant's toxic components, a number of antifungal
and natural pesticides have been made from it. For instance, elderberry leaves were laid near the heads of bedridden patients to keep
away flies.[31] The juice of the plant was used to ward off pests on
certain crops. The elder was also used to treat various ailments in
livestock, generally following the same principles for treating people.

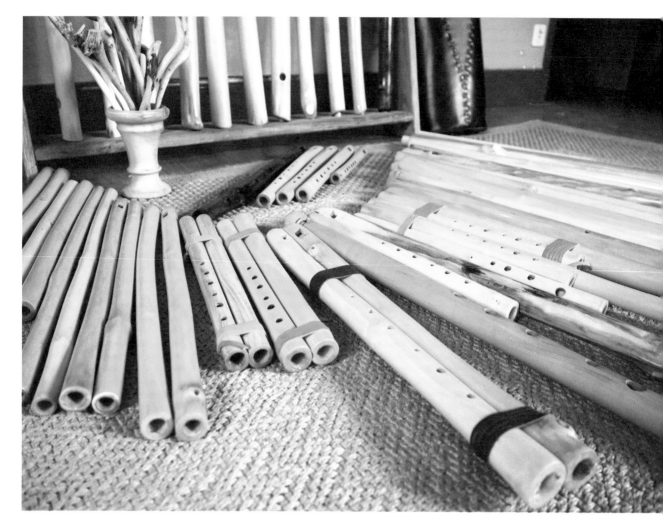

▲ An assortment of elder flutes in many styles and sizes. MAX BRUMBERG, BRUMBERG FLUTES

In the mid-1900s, elderberry, like many traditional foods, medicinals, and herbals, lost ground to the age of antibiotics. But one reason you picked up this book is because elderberry has regained so much ground over the past decade; interest in the plant is probably the highest it has been in a hundred years. So now that we are more familiar with elder's story, let's look at how to make it a part of ours.

well.

Oil of Elder Leaves

For the treatment of bruises, wounds, &c., take one part of the leaves of the common elderberry and three parts of good linseed oil, and boil gently till the leaves are quite crispy, and the oil is then pressed out and again heated with more leaves till it becomes quite green. This is much used by veterinary surgeons.

◀ Old books explore the use of elder for both people and animals. *WRINKLES AND NOTIONS FOR EVERY HOUSEHOLD*, 1890, ARCHIVE.ORG

Herbs and flowers. Levant wormseed, cloves, poplar, lavendar, elderberry, mullein, calendula, safflower, arnica, chamomile (Roman and German), insect flowers (Persian 10 and Dalmatian, cusso, lily-of-the-valley, Irish moss, Iceland moss, cannabis, clover, pulsatilla, adonis, broom, galega, melilot, eupatorium, grindelia, tansy, wormwood, mugwort, lobelia, peppermint, spearmint, marjoram, thyme, American pennyroyal, horehound, catnip, skull- 15 cap, chiretta, centaury, helianthemum, euphorbia pilulifera, drosera, verbena

◀ A page from the 1913 American Pharmacological Society Syllabus. ARCHIVE.ORG

Oil of Elder-flowers. *Syn.* WHITE OIL OF ELDER; OLEUM SAMBUCI ALBUM, O. SAMBUCINUM (P. Cod.), L. *Prep.* From the flowers, as OIL OF CHAMOMILE. Emollient and discussive.

Oil of Elder-leaves. *Syn.* GREEN OIL, GREEN OIL OF ELDER, OIL OF SWALLOWS; OLEUM VIRIDE, O. SAMBUCI VIRIDE, L. *Prep.* 1. Green elder leaves, 1 lb.; olive oil, 1 quart; boil gently until the leaves are crisp, press out the oil, and again heat it till it turns green.

2. As before, but by maceration, at a heat under 212° Fahr. More odorous than the last.

3. Elder leaves, 1 cwt.; linseed oil, 3 cwt.; as No. 1.

Obs. The last form is the one usually employed on the large scale. It is generally coloured with verdigris, ½ lb. to the cwt., just before putting it into the casks, and whilst still warm; as, without great skill and a very large quantity of leaves. the deep-green colour so much admired by the ignorant cannot be given to it. The oil is got from the leaves by allowing them to drain in the pan or boiler (with a cock at the bottom), kept well heated. Emollient; in great repute among the vulgar as a liniment, in a variety of affections.

◀ COOLEY'S CYCLOPAEDIA, 1880, ARCHIVE.ORG

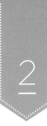

2

Description, Anatomy, Terminology, and Nutrition

DESCRIPTION AND ANATOMY

You will enjoy the elder far more if you take a little time to become familiar with its anatomy and the various terminology used to describe different parts of the plant.

First, what is the elder? It is a perennial, medium to large shrub or small tree, with large pinnately compound leaves; that is, leaves form in pairs on opposite sides of each stem. The elder produces flowers that turn into drupes in late summer through early fall.

Samuel Thayer gives an excellent description of elder, stating,

The leaf typically consists of seven leaflets, which are sharply serrated, 2–5 inches (5–13 cm) long, elliptic with sharply pointed tips, and sessile or growth on very short petioles. The leaves and stems of elderberry give off a strong, unpleasant odor when cut or bruised.

The small, white, five petaled flowers, about .25 inches (6 mm) across, are produced in rounded, somewhat flat top clusters called symes, at the ends of the branches. These cymes are typically 4–9 inches (10–23 cm) across, and each can contain hundreds of flowers. The fragrant blossoms open in the late June and July.[1]

It has a growth habit of around 5 to 12 feet in height, though in some locations much larger sizes are possible. Elder tend to grow in

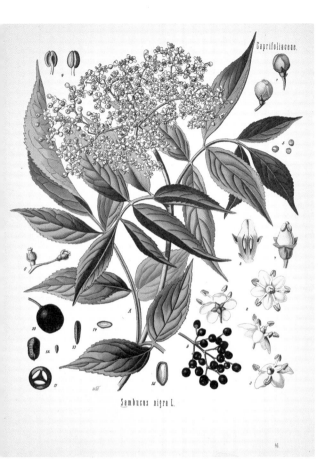

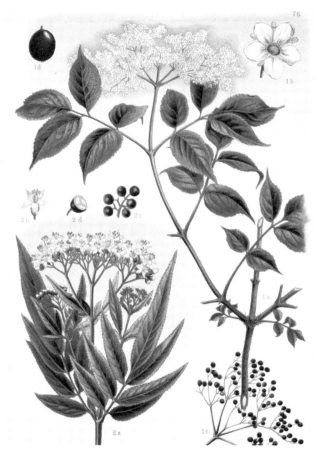

dense thickets, similar to blackberries and raspberries, since in the wild the plant reproduces by rhizomes and root suckers, as well as by seed.

The plant's fruit, while often called a berry, is technically a drupe. It starts out green and turns purplish to black when fully ripe. Elderberries make up for the small fruit size with tremendous production—each cyme may produce hundreds of berries. The small fruit size doesn't make harvest any harder, though. You can snip off the entire cyme, collecting dozens of berries at a time with ease.

The branches of the elderberry are semi-hollow and filled with pith. They are also quite pliable, bending over as the weight of the fruit clusters increases as harvest approaches. The older branches

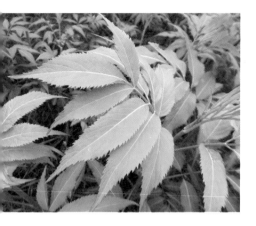

▲ Elder leaf.

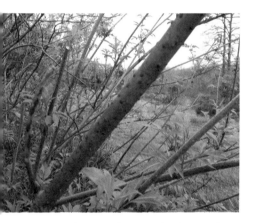

▲ Lenticels are one key feature of the elder that make it easy to differentiate from a few possible look-alikes when foraging.

are covered in lenticels, specialized tissues that allow the plant to breathe. These lenticels are a key feature to help you more easily identify elder when foraging.

The above description mainly applies to the American (*Sambucus canadensis*) and European (*Sambucus nigra*) elderberry. Generally speaking, when someone thinks or talks about elderberry, this is what they have in mind. Two others—the blue (*Sambucus cerulea*) and red (*Sambucus pubens*, *racemosa*, and *callicarpa*)—also are worth mentioning. The blue elder is similar to the American and European, but every facet of it is larger than its cousins. It will sometimes become a tree, reaching 40 feet high or more. Its range only slightly overlaps that of its smaller relative, mainly growing in British Columbia and through the western United States, especially the northwestern states and northern California. The berries are generally a blue color with a heavy white bloom on them.

The red's range overlaps with the blue, but is much, much wider—as far north as Alaska and across much of the northern half of the United States. It is in many ways unlike its cousins—ripening much earlier and having grape-like fruit clusters. The berries range from red to yellow orange and cannot be used or prepared like its black and blue cousins. It is also generally regarded as the least desirable to grow or forage, as the flavor is quite poor for such a vibrant and colorful fruit. Even the ripe berries are considered by all to be toxic.

TERMINOLOGY

If after reading all this, it seems a bit unclear or confusing, take a moment to review the definitions provided below. Especially when foraging, but also when tending a plant such as the elder, it is important to understand basic plant terminology to help ensure you don't collect from other commonly mistaken options.

- **Pinnation:** the arrangement of structures along a common axis, such as leaves along a branch or stem

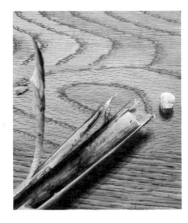

▲ Elder wood isn't hollow, but filled with a soft, easy to remove plant material called pith.

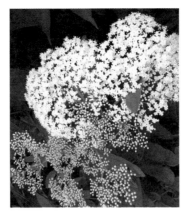

▲ The flowers of the elder are not just edible, but incredibly beautiful.

- **Petiole:** the part of a leaf that connects to the leaf base and the branch or stem of the plant

- **Pith:** a course, grainy vascular cell material found inside the stalks and branches of some plants

- **Lenticel:** a specialized tissue on certain plants that creates a pore through which the plant can directly exchange gases from internal tissues with the surrounding environment

- **Cyme:** a flower cluster with a central stem bearing a single terminal flower that develops first, the other flowers in the cluster developing as terminal buds of lateral stems.

- **Pedicel:** a short flower stalk in a bundle of flowers, grows off the main stem (peduncle). Also called an inflorescence.

- **Umbrel:** An inflorescence that has multiple pendicles that branch off from a common point on the peduncle

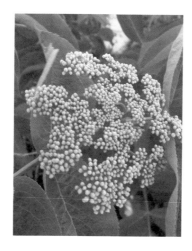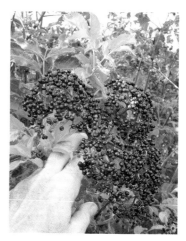

▲ The fruit of the elder starts green and slowly ripens over the summer.

- **Drupe (stone fruit):** similar to berries, elder berries are technically drupes (like apricots and almonds)

- **Root sucker:** a shoot (new plant) that springs forth from buds that form along a plant's root system. These allow propagation of some plants by removing the root sucker with some intact root structure.

- **Rhizome:** Greek for "mass of roots," a modified plant stem that grows horizontally underground, sending out both roots and shoots. Above-ground stems are called stolons.

BENEFITS AND STUDIES

Many people become interested in the elder because of its medicinal value, especially for dealing with the flu and colds. Such use is not only supported by history; modern studies have shown great promise to various preparations made from elderberries. Research has focused especially on the berries' ability to reduce the severity and symptoms of cold and flu. There are many reasons why elderberry helps our bodies deal with infection. Some studies show that phytochemicals (plant chemicals) found in the elderberry make it

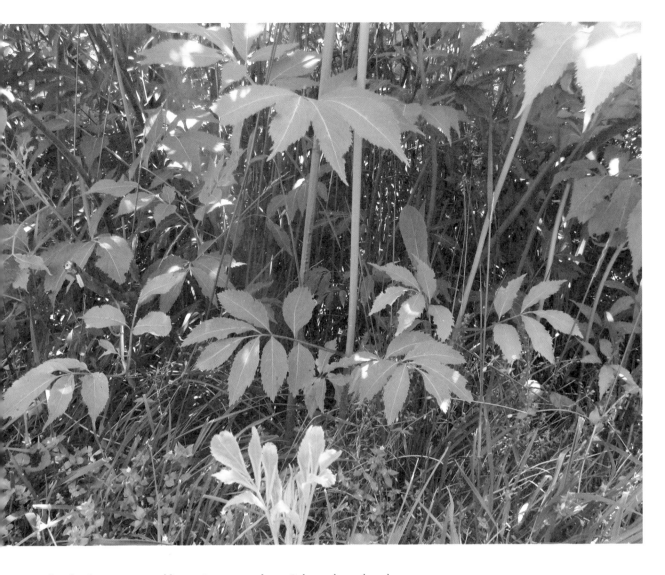

harder for viruses and bacteria to reproduce. Others show that they help marshall and bolster our immune system's performance. Elderberries show promising results in research involving inflammation and diabetes.[2]

NUTRITION

Elderberry is often called a "superfruit," an appellation well deserved for such a small food. It packs quite a bit into each berry![3] It is higher in many phytochemicals—especially flavonoids like anthocyanin—

than most any other berry. For instance, in terms of antioxidants, its ORAC (Oxygen Radical Absorbance Capacity) score is twice that of blueberries and 3½ times that of raspberries and strawberries.[4]

- Elderberries— 147
- Blueberries— 62
- Cranberries— 95
- Mulberries— 53
- Raspberries— 40
- Strawberries— 36

Elderberries are also higher in many minerals and other nutrients. These beneficial components are not alone, though. Elder also contains a wide range of possibly dangerous chemicals, such as alkaloids and glucosides. The elderberry plant's long history of medicinal use is tied to both its many beneficial and dangerous potent plant-based chemicals, from root to leaf to berry, and all parts in between.

Can I Eat Elderberries Raw?

There is a fair bit of debate over consuming raw elderberries. Some state that many if not all American cultivars are safe to consume raw, save the red, but none of the European.

I suggest people err on the side of caution and skip raw elderberries, especially until this debate is fully settled. It isn't like you can check a bush's ancestry easily when you come across it in the wild! While some people report being able to eat small to moderate amounts with no issues, some have reported mild to even severe nausea from consuming the fresh berries. Exactly why is not entirely clear. A recent research project by the University of Missouri found that ripe American elderberry cultivars' berries and seeds contained little to no glycosides, unlike European varieties. These cyanide-forming compounds are one reason the elder is so toxic in all its parts. Even so, some people still report significant stomach upset and other issues from consuming raw berries or raw juice from American elders. Either way, some people don't find the taste of fresh American elderberries overly appealing. The elderberry shines in the many traditional ways people prepared and used them, which generally involved cooking the berries to temperatures over 180°F (82°C) or fermentation that breaks down and deactivates the problematic chemicals.

If you do decide to try raw fresh berries, make sure that they are fully ripe, and limit yourself to a small quantity initially to see how you respond. If few of the berries have been picked by birds, that is probably a sign that the berries are not yet ready or otherwise are higher in defensive chemicals, and thus, move on to another bush or continue to wait for the berries to fully ripen.

For other parts of the plants, if used in food or as herbal preparations, make sure you consult appropriate guides, with all instructions, dosing recommendations, and warnings!

THE FAMILY DOCTOR.

Scurvey.

SARSAPARILLA, three ounces ; trefoil, one handful ; ground-ivy, one handful ; elderberry buds, one handful. Put them into three gallons of water, and boil them down to one-third. Take two drachm glassfuls before meat three times a day.

▲ *THE FAMILY DOCTOR, 18XX, ARCHIVE.ORG*

3

Cultivation and Care

ELDERBERRY ARE GENERALLY easy to grow and lovely to look at, which makes them a great addition to any home, homestead, or farm. Their habit allows for flexible use, even in urban or other restricted settings where you can grow them in plain sight as a part of most any kind of landscaping—even when other forms of productive and edible types of land use are prohibited! In this respect, it is similar to serviceberry and other edible landscaping plants that are usually unnoticed or overlooked by most people. Whether as a stand-alone plant or as a series of shrubs serving as a hedge or fence, elderberry does well in urban, suburban, or rural settings.

HOW TO CHOOSE AN ELDERBERRY VARIETY

There are several things to consider when choosing a particular type of elderberry to plant and propagate. The total number of cultivars now commercially available is over four dozen. Let's look at the main groups and differences in order to make a better decision about which ones you may want to try.

European versus American

The first major divide is between European and American species. For many decades, European and American elderberry were considered two different cultivars. More recent research and study now see

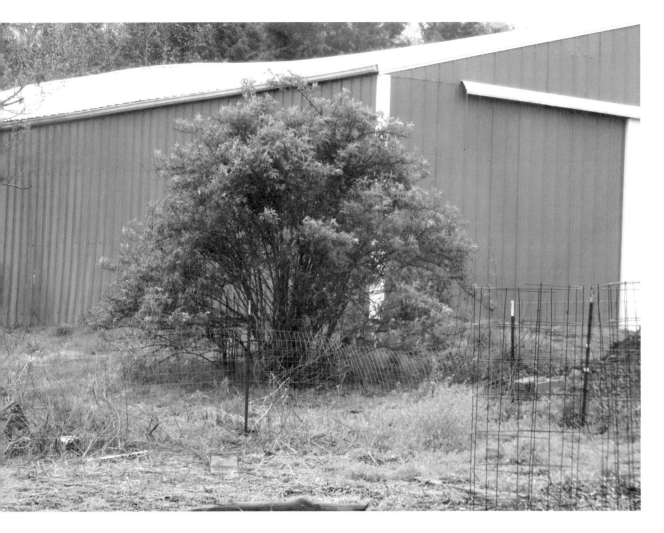

▲ Once a 6-inch hardwood cutting tucked into a marginal corner of our home-stead, this plant now towers some 14 feet tall.

the American variety as a subspecies of the European. This is mainly an academic rather than a practical issue.

Many European varieties do not perform well in the Midwestern United States, so choose cultivars carefully if going with European over American varieties.[1] Some particular growers have bred European varieties specifically for American soils and climates, so if you want to grow a European elder, I would suggest searching out and getting your plant stock from such a nursery.

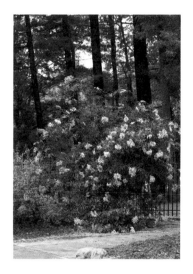

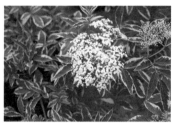

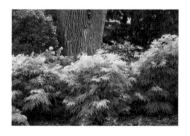

▲ Elder vary in appearance, habit, and production, so choose varieties that best meet your particular goals.

The main practical difference between the two is that the European varieties tend to produce larger fruit that is darker in color than American. Studies show that some American cultivars may be higher in some phytonutrients that may account for the difference in berry color, but at this point, there isn't enough research or data to make any firm conclusions.

Wild versus Domesticated

Often, someone will ask if they can just go out to the same place they forage elderberries and take cuttings or even remove a small section of the plant to establish on their farm or property. As long as you have permission from the landowner, of course you can!

Like the issue of European versus American, some of the differences between wild and cultivated elder are unclear. Generally, wild cultivars are less uniform in terms of fruiting and ripening, and also bring unknown resistance to certain pests and diseases. Wild cultivars may also be far more adapted to their particular ecosystem, and thus not take as well to relocation. Nutritionally or medicinally, there doesn't appear to be much evidence that wild have any advantage over cultivated varieties.

Ornamental versus Production

The next question when considering which elder to choose is do you want ornamental or production-oriented varieties? Some plants are bred specifically for looks, while others are bred for fruits. Some have greater aesthetic value, while others have greater production value. Realize, *all elder are both beautiful and productive*. It is a spectrum rather than a chasm that divides various options.

Some types are far more productive in terms of fruit. Others will still produce fruit, but their main value is in appearance, such as leaf color and shape. Ornamental cultivars will still produce fruit, but it is generally of a lesser quantity and/or quality than from those developed for fruit. In some situations, a more ornamental plant may be necessary, say to stay on the safe side of creating an edible landscape in areas that have strict rules against productive land use.

Hardiness, Shade Tolerance ·

The final consideration when choosing a cultivar is your location. Some varieties are more heat- and cold-tolerant than others, which is especially important if you live farther north or south. If you live toward the middle of the United States and not at exceptionally high or low elevation, almost all varieties are well suited for your climate.

Elder are somewhat shade-tolerant, though they will produce more and grow more vigorously if given part to full sun. Some varieties do show slightly greater shade tolerance, but this is another area that needs more research. As a final note, take information on recommended varieties, hardiness, and the like with a grain of salt. The performance of a particular type in one environment or place is no guarantee of how it will do at your place! Hence why I recommend you try at least three or four cultivars in a few different spots on your property and see which and where they do best for you.

AMERICAN VARIETIES	ZONE	GROWTH HABIT	NOTES
Adams	3-9	6-10 feet	Very similar to native elderberry, slightly larger berries
Black Lace	4-7	6-8 feet	Very distinctive leaves, not as good for berry production
Blue	3-10		
Bob Gordon	5-8		Discovered in 1999, very high yielding plant, early ripening Grows fruit on new canes
Ranch	3-9	5-7 feet	Compact variety, good yields
Wyldewood	4-8	5-8 feet	Known for its immense, almost foot wide flower heads
York	3-9	6-12 feet	Production variety—large berries and high yields per plant Becaue of height, also good for fencing
Marge	4-8	6-10 feet	Exceptional vigor and large berrries, along with nice upright habit. Created from European stock yet does exceptionally well in Midwest field trials.
EUROPEAN VARIETIES			
Samdal	3-7	6-8 feet	High-yielding clusters with smaller berries
Samyl	3-7	6-8 feet	Slightly higher yielding than Samdal
Black Beauty	4-7	5-6 feet	European import, distinctive dark leaves and pinkish blooms, more ornamental

The elderberry is one of the most widespread native plants on the North American continent. It is found from Florida to Nova Scotia, from New England to Manitoba, from Texas to the coastal Carolinas, and even as far south as northern Mexico. There are few places you cannot grow it, and generally, as long as you select a variety suitable for your location, it will grow well and rapidly.

Soil and Location Preferences

Elderberry is a hardy perennial plant. While it will do better in some situations and soils, it has thrived for thousands of years without human assistance in a wide range of terrains and territories. Native varieties are usually found along fencerows, hedgerows, sinkholes, streams, and other features that stop or block human machinery or otherwise go undisturbed by human activity. While elder prefers part to full sun, it also grows in partial shade, such as along wood lines.

Elder does well in most soil types, except those that are especially sandy. Such soils, since they drain well and rapidly, will need to be heavily amended with organic matter and possibly need significant supplemental irrigation for elder to perform well. Both muck and mineral soils produce fine elderberry bushes. Soil pH is of little concern unless your pH is extreme—the plants can handle ranges of 4.5 to 8.5, though a range of 5.5 to 7.5 is preferred.

Also note, because elderberry has an extensive root system, it is a useful plant to stabilize soils that are prone to erosion. Stream banks, pond and lake shores, along with any other erosion-prone sites are excellent candidates for elderberry, and often places that the plant establishes itself naturally.

Elderberry is an important food source for many species of birds—too many to list! It is also a fall food for many animals—the leaves are generally unpalatable in the springtime, but as summer wanes, the leaves sweeten, becoming an inviting food for deer, elk, goats, and many other browsers. Some will also eat the berries.

Because it is susceptible to *Verticillium* and tomato mosaic virus, avoid planting elder where or near mint, alfalfa, potato, or tomato grow or were recently grown.

Starting Your Elderberry Plants

If you have space and budget, do not limit yourself self to only one species of elder. We started with four cultivars and quickly realized that two of them did far better than the others, and one in particular towers above the rest. One practical benefit of growing more than one variety is the staggered blooming and harvest, providing more food for pollinators and people over the entire flowering season. I recommend you start with three or four varieties with three or more plants or cuttings of each. Plant these in two different spots for each type. Then see which do the best in your location, climate, and soil. In two to three years, you can then expand further after seeing which do best.

There is another important reason to plant more than one elderberry cultivar: you will see improved yields. While it's debatable whether some varieties of elderberry are self-fertile,[2] there is consensus that you will see improved yields if you plant more than one variety. So at the very least, you want a number of plants in relatively close proximity to one another for best results. Also note, some cultivars are more for aesthetics than production. This creates an opportunity to mix and match higher-yielding varieties with those of visual or other interest.

You may notice some peculiar results that, if you plan to expand your production or plantings, help you make better decisions about what bushes do best where on your land. For instance, one bush of ours in particular produces four times more berries than all the rest of our current production of ten bushes combined. This bush is a clear winner for further propagation for us. A different cultivar may perform far better for you.

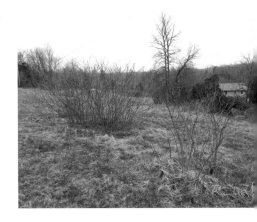

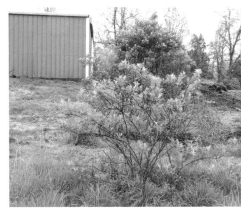

▲ Planting a few different varieties will let you see which do best on your property. These were all started at the same time, yet have grown and produced quite differently.

Spacing, Irrigation, and Fertilization

For spacing, the general recommendation is about 6 to 8 feet (2 to 2.6 meters) between plants, with rows spaced 8 to 12 feet apart (2.5 to 4 meters). Some varieties may benefit from slightly different spacing, so it is best to check, especially for ornamental or uncommon varieties. When you look at that little 5-inch or so elderberry cutting or plant in a pot, you may think, *Wow, does it really need this much space?* Yes, it does! In a few years, that little plant will take up 30 or more square feet! Also note, since elderberry are primarily wind pollinated, plant spacing and density are very important to yields. If they are too far apart or too sparsely planted, or located where your dominant wind patterns can't move pollen from plant to plant, your yields will suffer.

Note: If your goal is commercial production, the row and spacing recommendations change substantially. Here, rows are generally 10 to 12 feet apart to accommodate the equipment used in elderberry orchards, and plants in each row of a single cultivar are spaced 2 to 3 feet apart and pruned heavily to encourage maximum production.

Depending on the variety you choose and your goals, elder also make excellent living fences, hedgerows, or screens. These uses are noted back to the Greeks and Romans. So common was this use in England that they had this saying: "An elder stake and a blackthorn, either will make a hedge to last forever." When using elderberry for such purposes, you will need to consider and adjust both the varieties you choose and their spacing, along with how you plan to manage pruning.

If you are in a drier climate, the plants will benefit greatly from supplemental irrigation. Elders are not drought tolerant. Ideally, they should receive around 1.5 to 2 inches of rain or supplemental water per week, slightly more during unusually hot, windy, and dry conditions. While you can use a hose, sprinkler, or drip tape, watering stakes or spikes are preferred. Air watering is a common cause of many plant-borne diseases, and can help encourage powdery mildew among other problems for your plants.

For a long row of plants, drip irrigation also works very well. However, one problem is it provides water to weeds and other unwanted plants, so stakes or spikes are superior, given elder's low tolerance for weeds when first planted. What matters most is that the plants, if nature doesn't provide, get sufficient supplemental water. So, don't let the drawbacks of any method keep you from giving them what they need if that is what you have available.

While many elderberries do okay on relatively low-fertility soil, they will bear better with proper fertilization. It is best to test your soils before fertilizing or amending them. Most soils will benefit from the addition of compost, especially manure-based composts, before planting. As a general rule, you can fertilize bushes each year with a 10-10-10 product. Use ½ pound per plant per year of the plant's age, up to 3 pounds per plant. So, for a 4-year-old bush, use 2 pounds of fertilizer. Another excellent supplement for elderberry is fish emulsion—you can apply about ½ cup per plant diluted in water, either sprayed around the base of the plant or as a foliar feed to provide fertilization along with additional trace minerals and nutrients that standard fertilizers usually lack.

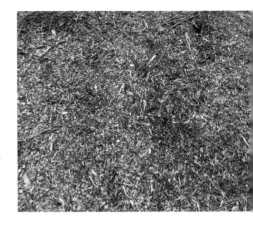

▲ A well-aged wood-chip or similar mulch will help new plants with both soil water retention and weed suppression.

Weeding and Mulching

As a perennial, elders do best with a light to moderate mulch that is 2 to 4 inches deep. An aged wood-chip or leaf-mold mulch is preferred, but straw or similar materials also work if you can't get your hands on the former. As with any plant, do not mound the mulch directly up against its base! Instead, leave a few inches of space in all directions. Mulch is especially helpful for elderberries, since they do best in moist soils, and mulches help keep the soil from drying out between rains or waterings. In very cold climates, mulch may also offer some protection from damage caused by extreme cold, especially when insulating snowfall is lacking.

Weeds can severely hamper elders during their first two years—the young plants do not compete well with weeds. Because the bushes are shallow rooted, hand weeding or any other tool that

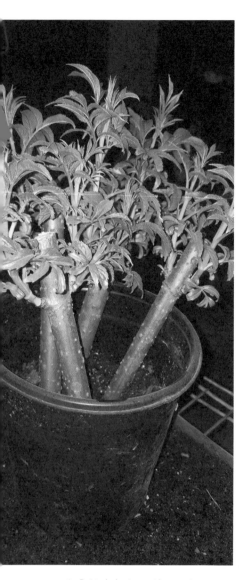

▲ Potted plants are the most expensive way to get an elder-berry—always inspect the plants for damage, disease, or root binding before buying!

CHERIE MCDIFFETT

doesn't cut into or disturb the soil is best. Especially during the first year, exercise great care so that you do not damage the developing root system. This is another benefit of mulch, as it reduces weed pressure and makes it far easier to remove weeds around new plantings without damaging them in the process. So plan to mulch your plants. Once established, they tend to suppress weeds themselves, but don't neglect to mulch even if it's not needed for weed suppression—it has many other benefits to your plants and the soil!

If you have multiple rows, the paths between them are also best put into mulches, either carbon based—wood chips, straw, and the like—or living ones, such as mixed clovers and other short plants that both build up the soil and are easy to maintain by mowing.

PURCHASING AND PROPAGATION

When first starting an elderberry patch or wanting to increase the number of plants on your property, there are several ways to go about it.

Purchasing Plants

Live plants are best purchased in the late winter or early spring and planted before high temperatures and dry conditions set in. If your soil or location is prone to drought, make sure you plan ahead so that you can provide water as needed. When you receive your plants, look them over to ensure they are healthy and undamaged. Keep them watered and in a cool, partially shady location until ready to transplant. Don't purchase plants that are overly large for their containers—if you do, make sure you get them into the ground as soon as possible.

When you remove them from their pots to transplant, take a moment to inspect their roots. They should be white to cream, some perhaps looking a little "fuzzy." If the roots are dense and spiraling against the outer edge of the container, the plant is root-bound. You will need to gently work all around the root ball to loosen the roots and encourage proper root growth after transplant. Root binding happens when a plant is kept in too small a pot for a long period of

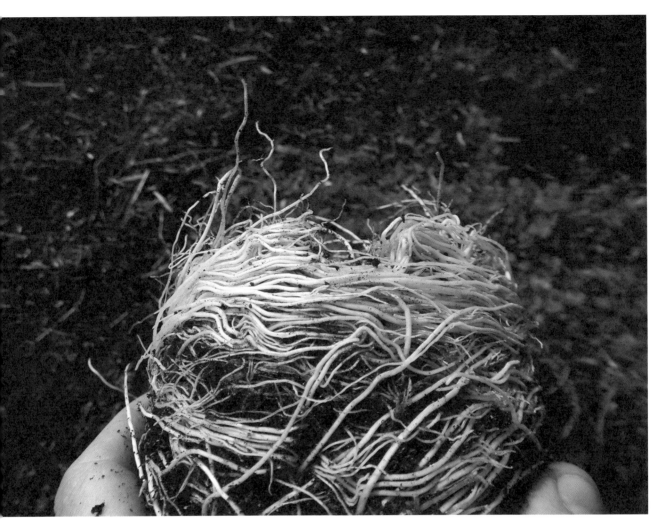

▲ While at first glance this plant has a healthy, extensive root system, it is also badly root-bound from long ago having outgrown its container.

time, so the best way to avoid the problem is getting the plants into the ground as soon as possible and using bigger pots to begin with so you have a larger window to get them out of the pots and into the ground without causing problems.

Depending on your starting soil, dig a hole approximately 12 to 18 inches deep and wide, and fill it with a rich humus soil/potting mix. You can add some compost, but don't overdo it with elder, as you want to encourage root formation, not foliage, the first year. So,

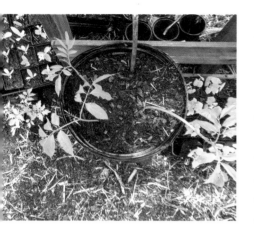

▲ Softwood cuttings are easy to take, but require proper conditions and care to create a viable transplant.

lots of nitrogen is not wanted. Plan to lightly water 2 to 3 times per week for 3 to 4 weeks until the plants are established, more if it is abnormally dry or warm.

Growing from Cuttings

Generally, elderberries are propagated through cuttings—4-to-8-inch segments of plant or wood that will root out if conditions are right—that create a new plant identical to the parent plant. This is somewhat similar to how potatoes and sweet potatoes work. You take a potato, cut it into pieces, plant it, and violà! You get many new potatoes, all genetically identical to the original.

Cuttings are far more affordable than live plants. Generally, a single live plant costs $20 to $30. For the same price, you can often get a dozen or so cuttings. They are also much easier to ship and far less likely to suffer damage during shipment, further reducing their cost. So, you can see why they are often the recommended way to plant and propagate!

Taking Your Own Cuttings

If you already have elderberry bushes, you can easily take your own cuttings either to sell or to expand your patch. A good pair of garden shears is really the only tool required. There are two major types of cuttings: softwood and hardwood. Their care and use differ somewhat, so we will cover each separately.

Softwood Cuttings

Softwood cuttings are done in the late spring through midsummer. These generally are best planted in the early fall, after they have had time to establish a strong root system for transplanting. Look for new young branches that are soft, just turning from green to brown, and are free of damage, disease, or the presence of pests.

Work your way down the branch, cutting it into 5-to-6-inch pieces. Some suggest cutting the top end flat and the rooting, lower side at an angle—this helps ensure you plant the cuttings correctly into the ground or pots. You can also seal the top with a food-grade wax to prevent disease. Remove all but the two topmost leaves from each segment. At this point, you can root the cuttings out in water or soil. I suggest sticking with the soil method whenever possible as it produces stronger, healthier roots for planting.

It is best to pot cuttings deeply—for a 4-to-6-inch cutting, 3 to 4 inches deep into an amended potting mix, either in pots or directly in the ground. Ensure that the soil stays moist. One drawback to softwood cuttings is that **they require misting from 2 to 4 times per day**. The plants take about 12 or more weeks to develop sufficient roots during this time as well. You should wait until the fall to transplant new softwood plants into the ground, and prune the plants before the first winter down to only about 2 to 4 inches of new growth.

Hardwood Cuttings

Hardwood cuttings are typically done in the late fall or early winter, when the bush is completely dormant. The process is similar to softwood cuttings, except these are relatively shelf stable if stored properly. So you can take a large number of cuttings in the winter and sit and wait on them until spring. If you want to plant in the spring or have plants to sell, hardwood cuttings are the way to go, since you can root them out over winter for spring transplanting and sales.

Take slightly longer cuttings for hardwood: 6-to-10-inch pieces. Each cutting should have one, preferably two, bud spots along its length.

Once ready to plant your hardwood cuttings, you will first need to soak them in well or distilled water for 24 hours. Regular tap water is not recommended because the chlorine and other chemicals it contains may negatively impact the cutting. After soaking, some suggest using rooting hormones, either synthetic (not permitted for certified organic or naturally grown operations) or natural ones, such as honey or willow bark water. Dip the cutting's lower end in Hormodin #1 rooting hormone or soak for 5 to 10 minutes in a willow tip or honey decoction. The decoctions can be stored for many months, or willow

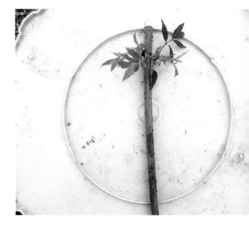

▲ Hardwood cuttings are the easiest and most affordable way to start or propagate elder.

tips can be harvested and dried for winter use. Then, put the cuttings either into a transplanting bed, pot, or directly into the ground. If in a transplanting bed, give each cutting around 6 inches in all directions for root development.

Care for Cuttings

It is imperative that the soil stays moist for both types of cuttings and that they are kept in a cool, shady location until well established. A basement, garage, or, ideally, a sheltered, shady outdoor location all work. The plants root best at temperatures between 36° to 46°F (2° to 8°C). Warmer temperatures encourage the formation of foliage.

One method that can help is to "tent" the cuttings, which traps moisture and raises the humidity. Be careful—tents exposed to sunlight become miniature greenhouses, encouraging leaf growth instead of root formation and can easily cook young plants in just a few hours if left unattended. The problem with excessive leaf growth is the plant won't have sufficient roots to support the foliage and also lacks sufficient reserves to successfully form both. So try and keep the plants as cool and semi-shaded as possible for their first 8 to 12 weeks.

Replanting Runners and Taking Root Cuttings

Another easy method is to take advantage of the elder's desire to reproduce by runners. The best time to propagate by replanting a runner is during late fall or early winter, when the plant is completely dormant. In the spring, when new plants pop up around a main trunk, put down a flag next to the new growth to mark it for winter relocation. Dig about 4 inches all around, and prune the top growth down to 4 to 6 inches. You can then put these either into 6-inch (1-gallon) pots or directly into their new home. If directly replanting, mulch the soil around the plant.

If in pots, keep them in a place sheltered from winds. In very cold climates, it may be best to keep them out of freezing temperatures or bring them into a sheltered location, such as barn, high tunnel, cold basement or garage. If you bring them indoors, make sure that they don't dry out! Every 1 to 2 weeks, lightly water the soil to keep it moist.

Root cuttings—digging up pieces of root and then replanting them—is also an easy way to create more plants. Since elder roots tend to grow shallowly along the ground, they are easy to dig and collect. Look for pencil-size or slightly larger roots, about 4 to 6 inches long, that have one or more nodes. Lay the cutting horizontally in a container and cover with about ¾ to 1 inch of light soil or potting mix. Keep moist and warm—these will often produce 2 to 3 new plants per cutting that can then transplant into the ground come fall.

Seeds

Less common, but still possible, is propagation via planting seeds collected from the berries. The reason this is less common is that while the plants produce a prodigious amount of seeds—2 to 5 per berry, so many thousands per plant—the seeds need a long period of stratification before sprouting. What is stratification? Many perennial plant seeds need to undergo a long period of cold, dark, moist conditions before they break out of their dormancy and germinate.

For elder, you can place seeds in a shallow, ½-inch or so, dish containing sand or vermiculite. Make sure the medium is moist. Cover the dish and place it in a cold fridge—ideally just above freezing, around 34° to 38°F (1° to 3°C). The seeds should stay in the fridge for around 2 months. When spring comes, place the trays outside in a partially shady place and ensure the soil stays moist. Hopefully in a month or so you will see little elder sproutlings pop up from the soil![3]

Given the ease of other propagation methods detailed above, you can see why few employ this particular route. The one benefit? You may end up with new and unique cultivars. Seed production is the main way new varieties arise, as it is the only method of propagation that introduces genetic chance into the equation. You may also end up with total duds! Also, a final note on seeds and seedlings: unlike cuttings, it takes an additional year to get to fruit production. So instead of 2 years, it generally takes 3 before you will see fruit set.

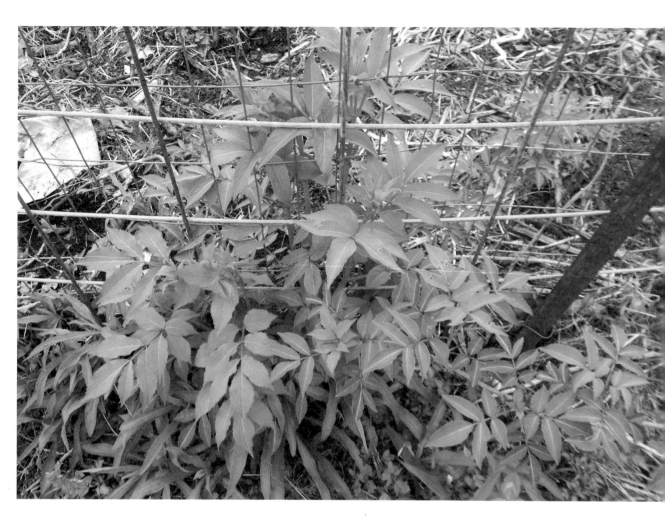

▲ This little baby elder popped up about 10 yards from its parent plant along a fence line nearby, probably deposited by a bird or a young boy who lost track of a berry. Note, even when young, the distinctive leaf shape and lenticels all along the bark.

If you try this approach, I recommended starting the seeds in larger cell count trays, such as 48s, and put 2 seeds per cell. Then, transplant successful seeds into larger cells as needed.

FIRST THREE YEARS OF GROWTH AND FRUITING

"Sleeps, creeps, then leaps." Many perennials follow this growing pattern. The first year, most of their time and energy goes into establishing a strong root system. The second year, you will get good growth and a modest fruit crop. The year after, your plants will grow and expand vigorously. This is why proper spacing is important for your elder starts—while small at first, each will eventually expand with exceptional vigor and need a great deal of space!

Elders sometimes produce flowers and thus fruit during their first year. With some perennials, it is usually recommended that you remove the blossoms to prevent fruiting during the first 2 years. This encourages and enables the plant to put its limited resources into growing roots and foliage, instead of putting it into fruit that then is removed from the plant. Consider it a short-term loss for a much longer-term gain. With elderberry, since the blossoms are highly prized for making wine, cordials, fritters, and many other things, it really isn't a loss at all if you collect them the first year and wait until the second or third for fruit.

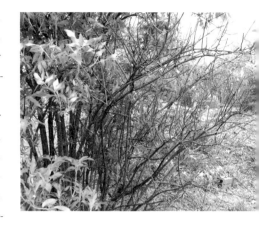

▲ Pruning takes just a little time each year to ensure your plants stay healthy and productive. This elder has a damaged or diseased section that needs to be examined and removed.

CARE AND PRUNING

To prune or not to prune, that is the question! Now, realize, in nature, elderberry goes unpruned, save by the action of animals, insects, disease, or intense weather. This doesn't mean we shouldn't prune our plants, just that it is not absolutely necessary. For landscaping purposes, when space is limited, and for maximum production, pruning is very important. It also has a number of benefits—better plant health, easier harvest, and increased yields to name a few. Also note, no one approach to pruning applies to all elderberries. Some cultivars have well-defined central trunks, while others do not. Some have a more upright, tree-like growth habit, some more shrub- or hedge-like. So you will need to adjust and adapt to the particular varieties you plant.

Ground Pruning

One approach to elderberry pruning involves reducing the plants to ground level, generally via some type of mowing during winter. The plants then rapidly regenerate from the crown or root suckers the following spring.

Studies show that such an approach has three main benefits:

· fruit and plant height are lower and uniform, making harvest easier and faster.
· ripening and harvest window is reduced, reducing labor and loss.
· fewer and larger cymes, so while the yield per plant may not be higher, the size of clusters is larger but the number fewer, resulting in less labor and faster harvest.

At the same time, a few people have reported that, after ground pruning their patch, it became unproductive the next year, even with substantial regrowth of the bushes. This is because ground pruning only works with varieties that produce fruit on first-year canes/growth. So, you must be absolutely sure your variety is adapted for this method of pruning and well enough established—at least 3 to 4 years old—to regenerate quickly the following season.

Selective Pruning

A second way to prune shrubs and bushes is to selectively cut back branches, not only to remove damaged, broken, dead, or diseased portions of the plant but also to control or create a particular size and shape. All branches over 3 years old are candidates for pruning and removal—they become significantly less productive.

This is normally done using hand pruners and takes about 15 to 20 minutes per shrub.

Uniform Pruning

In between those two approaches, uniform pruning ignores the age of canes and instead cuts the entire bush to about 30 to 36 inches tall (1 meter). This approach is faster than selective pruning. It also lends itself to mechanization if you have a large number of bushes.

For all approaches, pruning should take place in the winter, generally mid- to late winter when the bushes are fully dormant.

What to do with all the waste wood from pruning? Many pieces should be suitable for all sorts of crafts that we discuss later in the book. The rest makes an excellent mulch or addition to your compost pile. Note that if your plants show any sign of pest or disease issues, it is best to use any mulch or compost you make from the pruned wood for other plants and purposes than your elderberry patch. Also, depending on the disease or pest, you may need to exercise care with other crops that are subject to the same diseases. You don't want to spread diseases or pests to your healthy plants, elderberry or others! For this reason, some growers will burn any infected or pest-ridden material.

PESTS AND DISEASES

Since elderberry is toxic and still mostly a wild plant, it tends to have excellent resistance to most pests and diseases. Few things will eat the plants, especially before fall, though a number of creatures will go after the ripe berries. Extracts from elderberry leaves are used to make insect repellant and to treat fungal infections such as powdery mildew and leaf spot—a reminder that a well-tended plant should result in a healthy plant!

Pests

A few key pest species may attack your elderberry, and thus you need to be able to identify them and know the proper treatment, if any, for each.

Japanese Beetles

Japanese beetles can sometimes afflict elderberry bushes. In our experience, this is more likely if attractive food sources—like raspberries, hazelnuts, pole beans, or other favorites—are in close proximity. The beetles will move or spread from the more common food source to the adjoining elderberry plants as they multiply and search for additional food supplies.

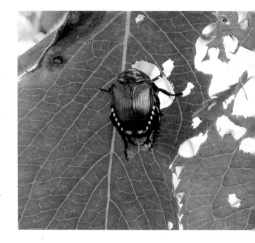

▲ Our most common elderberry adversary, Japanese beetles, often spread to elderberry from other plants in adjoining growing spaces.

Handpicking into a bucket of water and then feeding to chickens or ducks is a great way to deal with the beetles for those managing small patches (10 to 20 bushes) comprising shorter bushes (8 feet tall and under). This is best done in the morning when the beetles are less active and alert. We use a 1-to-2-gallon pail or bucket filled with just a few inches of water. Look for leaves where the beetles are perched, and gently grab a foot or back on the branch. Shake the branch with the bucket held under the leaves and watch the beetles go plop.

If the infestation is too great or the patch too large, pheromone traps may be necessary. Beneficial nematodes can also help by killing the beetles during the larval soil stage of their reproductive cycle. You can purchase these online to apply in either the early fall or spring. Just make sure that you purchase from a reputable supplier and acquire appropriate strains for the particular beetles and other pests you are trying to control.

If you have a dozen or more bushes, the use of an organic insecticide, usually neem or pyrethrin based, may be necessary for bad infestations. New technologies involving the use of super-heated air are also available in some areas. These show great promise for treating pests on many berry crops, including elderberry.

What to look for: damaged and bug-eaten leaves, presence of beetle droppings on foliage, presence of beetles.

What to do: hand collect into a bucket of water during heat of the day when beetles are less active and easy to capture, use of pheromone traps for bad infestations, apply beneficial nematodes in fall to reduce subsequent year populations.

Spotted Wing Drosophila

Spotted Wing Drosophila (SWD) is a small (approximately 3 millimeters) fly, often referred to as a vinegar fly because of its attraction to the smell of acidic fermenting things. The fly is non-native to the

United States and Canada, most likely brought via fruit imports from its native Asia. The pest is especially problematic because it damages fruit while still on the plant, not only when the fruit is overripe or otherwise decomposing, like most other vinegar flies.

This pest appears mainly limited to more northern regions currently, such as Minnesota, Michigan, and Wisconsin. Don't let their more northernly tendency lull you into complacency—they are present as far south as Kentucky and in many states in the North East. SWD impacts not just elderberry but a host of berry and fruit plants, including raspberry, blackberry, blueberry, and grape.

The good news? SWD is easy to control organically. Similar to a trap we have used inside for fruit flies and outdoors for flies, you can make your own very low-cost SWD traps out of almost any plastic jug—milk, soda, or other—and kombucha or a similar acidic beverage.

I find it very fitting that you can protect elderberry, which makes a lovely addition to kombucha, with the same beverage.

"To make the bottle trap, cut the top of a two-liter bottle so that you have an opening 3.5 cm in diameter. Push the top of the bottle into the interior of the bottle, until the cut edge is 6 cm on the inside of the trap. Cut the bottle 6 cm from the bottom. Take the bottom portion of the bottle, and using a hole punch, make two holes on opposite sides. These holes will be used for hanging the trap on a string. Insert a 50 cm length of string through the holes, and tie a 2 cm length of small diameter dowel to each end of the string. When using this trap, partially fill the bait reservoir with kombucha or a 60:40 mixture of red wine and vinegar. Insert what used to be the bottom of the bottle into the top of the trap, so that there is only about a 1 to 2 cm space between the opening into the trap, and the 'ceiling' of the space inside the trap. Use tape of any sort to hold the two parts together, and hang the string over a branch of a blueberry or raspberry plant so that the trap will mostly be kept in the shade. The upper part of the trap will form a second reservoir that may retained rain water, which may improve attraction of SWD to the trap."[5]

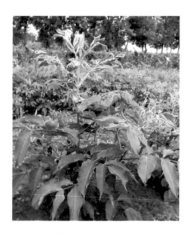

▲ You won't see these mites with the naked eye, but you may see their damage!

Note that you should combine trapping with other controls, such as ensuring adjoining habitat favor SWD predators and don't provide favorable conditions for their multiplication.

Also, a number of organic approved insecticides—PyGanic, Entrust, and neem oil—will also help control SWD. Even though these are organic, they may adversely impact other insects, including many kinds of beneficials. So if you use such controls, use them carefully and according to directions.

Eriophyid Mite

This microscopic mite comes in hundreds of host-specific species. If you have that, you won't see them! For this reason, the damage they do is often confused with herbicide drift or scorch—curled leaves, blistered leaves and bark, and sometimes galls. These carrot-shaped miniature mayhem makers are visible only under a microscope with 20x power. Not all parts of the country have significant mite pressure currently, though Missouri and some other Midwestern states do have some significant trouble spots.

What to look for: leaf curl and blister, galls

What to do: plant mite-resistant varieties, remove and dispose of old or damaged plant material by burning

If you have issues with mites, there are a few ways to try and control them. First, select resistant varieties when possible. Second, purchase predator mites to apply to the plants. You can also use organic insecticides, such as neem. Note that spring is the best time to spray for the mites because once they get reproducing, they do so rapidly. Also, generally speaking, a single round of spraying will not sufficiently control the mites—so plan to do one or two follow-up applications in another 7 to 10 days. Since most mite controls will also wipe out predatory mites and other beneficial insects, reserve them for only if the problem is quite severe. Instead, use pruning and removal of infested plant material as much as possible.[6]

Birds

Many species of birds love elderberries. For us, unless their foraging is extremely selfish, we don't mind sharing. Letting them eat some berries has an added benefit—they help spread and start new bushes! One of the main ways to ensure birds don't overly bother your crops is by having a diverse, healthy ecosystem that provides many other more attractive food resources for them to also enjoy. Generally, if you do that, their take of the elderberries will be tolerable.

If for some reason the birds are pilfering too much of the harvest or otherwise causing issues because of excessive droppings or damage to the bushes, netting is probably the best choice to protect the ripening fruit post-pollination. It is best applied after pollination, once fruit has set. You can also employ other bird deterrents.

Deer

Deer and similar browsers will consume the elders' foliage, some only in the fall as it sweetens, but some may also consume it early season or at any time. Some may also develop a liking for the berries. Deer are also a problem because of their rubbing, which can damage and even break branches off the plants. Ever have an itch you can't scratch? At the spot between their head and antlers, deer do! So, they look for smaller-diameter trees and shrubs to use as scratching sticks. This can cause significant damage to young trees or other plants because the rubbing removes the bark and then begins to damage the core.

You may need to employ dogs, fencing, hunting, or other forms of protection if deer are causing significant damage to your elderberry bushes. Trained dogs are an especially cost-effective deterrent for protecting not just your elderberries but many other susceptible crops. One or two dogs can keep 1 to 2 acres relatively free of deer damage if trained and managed well.

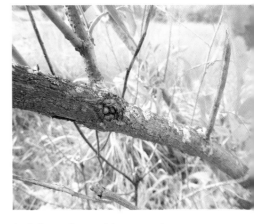

▲ Galls are abnormal tissue growths on leaves, stems, and other plant parts.

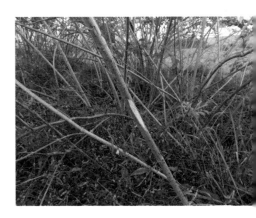

▲ Deer can do many kinds of damage to elderberry, including using it to deal with their itchy antlers.

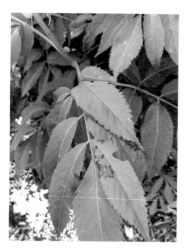

▲ Bacterial leaf spot.

Domesticated Livestock

Most domesticated livestock will generally not munch on foliage or other parts of elderberry. It is still best to exclude them from access, except maybe cows or sheep who make great lawn mowers between rows of bushes. Such a silvo-pasture approach to elderberries shows great promise, but requires good livestock management skills to ensure no damage befalls either the bushes or the livestock.

The only exceptions are pigs and goats. Pigs' rooting instincts make them very dangerous to the shallow root systems of elder bushes. Remember, goats will eat pretty much from tin cans to car tires. They tend to go after elderberry when they lack other better food sources, or when they have complementary food sources that allow them to safely consume elderberry and readily detox its more dangerous components. While you may be able to train goats to forego damaging your plants, I wouldn't trust them for a minute, and instead let them do what they do best—keep such shrubby and bushy plant material in check around other parts of your homestead or farm.

Diseases

Elderberry is susceptible to a few different diseases. If you are able to get certified disease-free root stock, this goes a long way to ensuring the health of your plants. Adequate water and proper nutrition also help prevent disease issues.

Generally, if a portion of a plant shows significant disease problems, it should be pruned and burned, or the entire plant pulled and burned.

Tomato Ringspot Virus

The most serious threat to elderberry, this virus, which is spread through soilborne nematodes, weakens and eventually kills plants. If you have had issues with this affecting other plants and want to try elderberry, make sure to plant it as far away as possible from any areas that showed evidence of the disease. You can also have your soil tested for it, but such testing is somewhat expensive.

Currently, there is no treatment or cure if a plant falls prey to this disease. Prevention through good practices is the priority. Beneficial nematodes for a few years before planting may also help with prevention.

Powdery Mildew

Good management is key. First, water by stakes, soaker hose, drip irrigation, or similar methods that do not drench the entire plant, especially the foliage. Make sure plants have sufficient space and proper air circulation, if needed, through aggressive pruning. Remove any affected leaves and other plant material and dispose of by burning.

Puccinia or Rust

This fungus affects both European and American cultivars, along with plants in the sedge family. Both plants are required for the fungi's life cycle. Orange lesions or pustules will form on the foliage of infected elder in spring, leading to deformation and possible defoliation if severe. Rust may also form on the cymes, leading to deformed and lost fruit. It is best to remove sedge before elder are planted, as once established among elder, it is difficult to impossible to remove. Neem applied in early spring may help impacted plants.

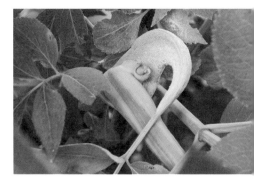

▲ Severe rust on an elder.
CHRISTOPHER LANDSEE, PRIMOCULTURE FARMS

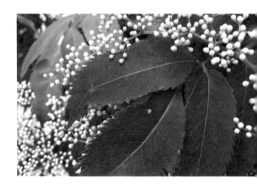

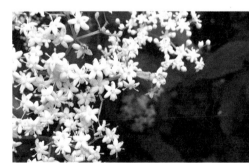

Early stage rust shows up as small dots on leaves and flowers, along with other plant parts. Remove as early as possible and dispose of infected plant materials by burning.

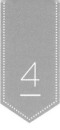

Harvesting, Foraging, and Preserving

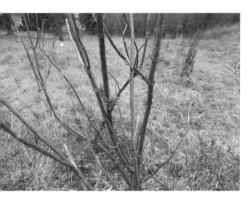

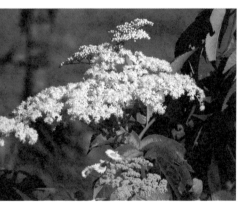

▲ CHRISTOPHER LANDSEE, PRIMOCULTURE FARMS

ELDERBERRY PLANTS go through three distinct stages each growing season.

Budbreak: Generally in February through March, the joints along branches where new growth and fruit form will break from their winter slumber and begin to grow.

Blossoming: In mid-May through June, blossoms will form.

Fruit set and ripening: From July all the way into September, fruit will set and ripen.

The window for harvest varies by around 6 to 8 weeks by location and cultivar in question, so it is important to learn to recognize when a good window for harvest has arrived in your area. Also, some of the most commonly mistaken plants have very different life cycles than elderberry, so knowing the elder's general habit in your area helps ensure you won't forage the wrong food!

For example, on our farm, a few groups ripen 2 to 4 weeks before the others. The native plants tend to ripen another week or so after our later groups. Also note, a particular mild winter and spring may shift your usual harvesting and foraging windows. As I sit here typing, our bushes are already in budbreak the first week of March

54 •

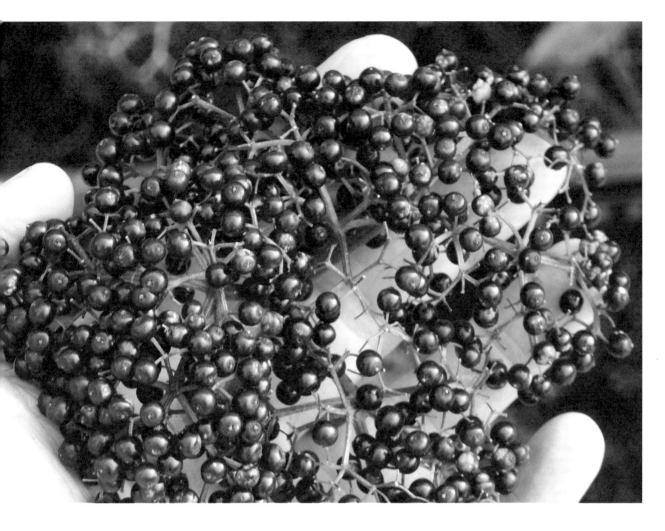

because of a mild late January and February. This may well shift out harvest 2 or 3 weeks this year! So it is best to check on your bushes throughout the season, especially during atypical years.

DANGEROUS AND OTHER LOOK-ALIKES

The story goes that the Canadian Mounties, in order to easily detect fake money, first and extensively study *the real thing*. When it comes to foraging, this is the best defense against making a bad mistake: know the plant you are foraging well first. If you know the elder well, you will quickly and easily distinguish it from the closest look-alikes, even if you don't know what they are.

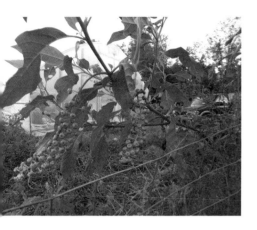

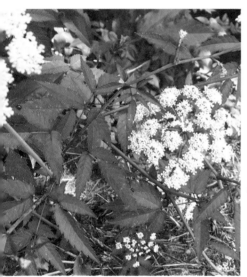

As a shortcut, it can help to know plants that are similar to elderberry that also grow in your area/region, and thus that you may mistake for the elder. Note, this list is not exhaustive, which is why it is crucial to learn the elder well. We will cover the plants that are most commonly mistook for the elder.

Poke

While poke does not look almost anything like elderberry, it is one of the more common plants people confuse with it. Unlike elderberry, poke will produce fruit across a much larger window of the growing season and has a much different leaf, stalk, and flower structure. The berries are much larger as well. Usually, poke is only mistaken for elderberry by people very new to foraging or plant identification.

Water Hemlock

Water hemlock (*maculata*) is one plant that more closely resembles elderberry. It is also quite dangerous, having the distinction of being "the most poisonous plant in the North Temperate Zone."[1]

There are a number of clues to help you not confuse the two, including:

- **Location:** Water hemlock, as the name implies, enjoys wet growing environments, and while its habitat overlaps with elder's, it is generally confined to more limited areas. You will find it close to creeks, streams, and similar water features, and it will even grow in water, a place elder cannot.

- **Stems:** Water hemlock is a herbaceous (not woody) plant. The stems are greenish in color and fibrous, instead of bark-covered and woody like trees and bushes. They contain no pith and also lack the distinctive lenticels of the elder.

- **Leaves:** While similar to the elder, they are not the same, as the veins end in the notches instead of the tips of the leaflets. On the elder, they tend to fade out or terminate at the tip of the teeth.

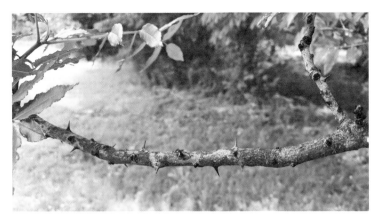

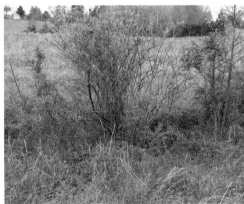

Aralia Spinosa (Hercules' club or Devil's Walking Stick)

The flowers and berries of Hercules' club do bear some resemblance to those of elderberry. Also, they have a long history of medicinal use, primarily for tooth pain. This plant presents a quick and easy way to differentiate it from elderberry: the main stalk will have thorns, which is why the plant has its peculiar name.

WHERE TO FORAGE

Elder occur in many different places. Generally speaking, they like moist areas, so along streams, spillways, lower areas of fence and tree lines, and similar spots are good places to look. In our area, almost every sinkhole contains one or more elderberry since water tends to run to the sinkholes and tractors can't mow or hay close to them. Many roads and tree lines may also have bushes usually just beyond the reach of the mowing crews.

Since they often occur along roads and other areas where property lines and land ownership may be unclear, I suggest it is best to ask the landowner for permission to collect from the bushes. On public lands, make sure you check if the place has any rules that may impact what and how much you may forage. Follow the rule of three when foraging: take at most ⅓ of any foraged food you collect, leaving ⅓ for others and ⅓ for animals and to provide plants for the future.

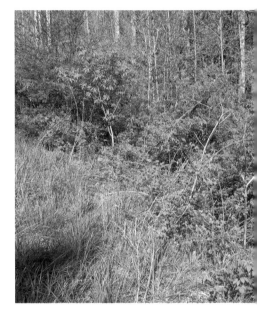

▲ Elder are often found along old fence and property lines, drives, roads, tree lines, and similar transitional spaces where woods, pasture, and other landscape features change.
CHERIE MCDIFFETT, RUSTIC ACRES FARM

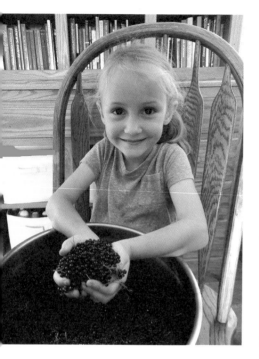

When to Harvest

In our region, elderberries are usually ready to harvest from mid-July to mid-August. Each region tends to have a specific window, so become familiar with yours—it is one time of year you don't want to miss! Elder give a simple visual cue, even from far away, when they are ready to harvest. For most types, the clusters of berries will droop down and the branches they are on will lean over as they ripen because of the increasing weight of the fruit.

Many factors determine when a specific bush's berries will be ready, such as the particular cultivar and the location. Even on the same bush, not all the clusters may ripen at the same time, so we harvest over the course of a few weeks. The general recommendation is to harvest 2 to 3 times, every 5 to 7 days, collecting the ripe clusters at each harvest.

A cluster is ready for harvest if 95 percent or more of the berries are fully ripe—plump and dark purple to black. While this means you may end up with a few underripe berries, we have found that if we wait until the entire cluster is fully ripe, we lose many to birds or drop, or if a storm or some other strong weather moves through, to wind and the heavy rain before we can harvest. So take the forecast into consideration with your collection schedule. It is best to avoid collecting any bunches that have clearly unripe green berries.

Elderberries, like most fruits and vegetables, are best harvested in the morning, after the dew has dried off but before the heat and strong sun reduce their moisture content. The peduncles, as long as they have received rain or irrigation, are nicely engorged in the morning, making harvest much easier. This is a more comfortable time of day to do such work and ensures the best-quality berries.

How to Harvest

Because elderberries grow in clusters, the fruit is easy to collect. We use pruning shears to remove entire clusters, placing them into a cloth-lined bin. Generally, we can collect about 20 pounds an hour.

How you manage your bushes will determine how difficult and labor-intensive harvesting is. A team of 2 or 3 people can quickly harvest a number of bushes, especially if they are kept pruned to around 6 feet or under.

We will reach back to where a branch and umbel meet, cutting on the umbel side an inch or so from the branch and dropping the entire cluster into the collection basket. Elderberry is a rather pliable wood, so for taller branches, we will gently bend the stalks until the clusters are within easier reach. If you have allowed your bushes to grow tall, a plant hook is the best way to reach higher branches and their berries.

On occasion, a cluster may have been visited by the back end of a bird or other animal. We generally discard or ignore any berries that have any bird or other animal droppings or show any signs of disease. They will possibly become new plants that we can then harvest or transplant come next year or the year after if they germinate.

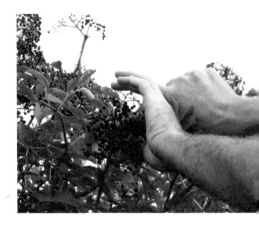

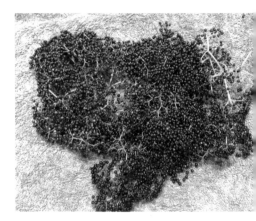

▲ A few simple tools make harvesting berry clusters easy, and kids of all ages are able to help harvest and clean your haul.

PRESERVING

Now that you have collected your elderberries, what will you do with them?

Elderberries are easy to preserve. Note that they don't keep well at room temperature once picked; within a day or so, they will degrade substantially in quality. Depending on your equipment and space, you can prepare them for later use in numerous ways. Also, you don't have to preserve elderberries before using them. Fresh elderberries can be used to make syrup, jelly, and many other things right off the bush!

It is mostly a matter of convenience and amount. Since we will collect 100 or more pounds of berries in just a few weeks—at a time of year that is far from cold and flu season—we tend to preserve the berries for the fall and winter. If you are primarily making shelf-stable creations from your elder bushes' beneficence, you may not need to prepare the berries for storage.

General Yield Information

What if you want to make a few gallons of elderberry wine? Or your family needs 10 bottles of elderberry syrup to get you through the winter? How many pounds of fresh berries should you aim to harvest? Let's look at some general yield data to help us plan how much and how to use our berries!

Elderberries are approximately 70 to 80 percent liquid. The following list shows the approximate amounts of berries and juice needed for some common products.

- 6 to 8 pounds of fresh berries makes 1 pound of dried elderberries
- 10 to 14 pounds of fresh berries makes 1 gallon of elderberry juice
- 2½ to 3½ pounds of fresh berries makes 1 quart of elderberry juice
- 1 pound of dried elderberries makes 8 16-ounce bottles of elderberry syrup
- 1 quart of elderberry juice makes 5 to 6 8-ounce jars of jelly

Dehydrating

The first time we preserved elderberries, it was completely by accident. While bike riding, the kids and I foraged some elderberries from along a fence line not far from our homestead, carrying them home in our T-shirts that we tied into bags on our handlebars. Once home, we placed the clusters in a bowl on top of our toaster oven. A few days later, my daughter exclaimed that the elderberries were nicely dehydrated (we use the toaster oven a lot during the summer!). Such an approach isn't too far off how the Native Americans dehydrated berries like the elder, setting them on warm, sunny rock exposures.

Almost any dehydrator will work, and if you have a gas oven and a house with relatively low humidity, you can sometimes even dry them in trays in the oven using just the heat from the pilot light. Start by rinsing the berries and letting them drip-dry for a few minutes on a clean towel. Then, arrange the clusters on the drying trays. You can either remove the berries or leave them on the umbels to dehydrate.

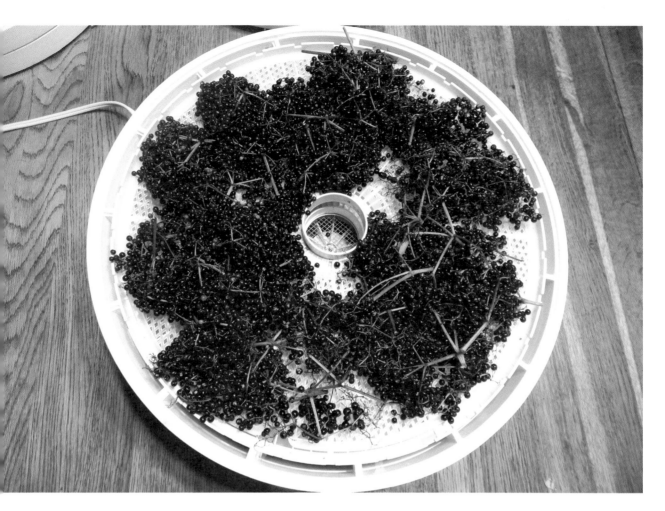

We prefer leaving them on, as the dried berries are easier to separate and less messy to deal with than the fresh.

The time required to dehydrate the berries depends on your machine and the temperature you use for drying, along with the ambient humidity. We generally dehydrate at about 140°F (60°C) for 12 to 18 hours. Since elderberries are small, they have a higher surface area to volume ratio than many other fruits, so they tend to dehydrate quickly. Once they are dehydrated, we will place the whole cluster in a storage bag and shake to make the berries come loose, using our hands or a large toothcomb to remove any stragglers. Place the berries in an airtight container or storage bag. Dried elderberries will last about 6 to 10 months stored in a cool, dry, dark place.

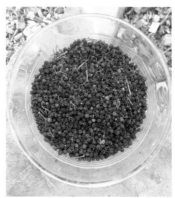

▲ Dehydrating is an age-old approach to preserving elderberries.

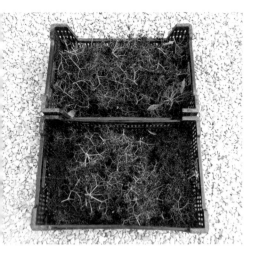

If you are in a place with sufficient breeze, sunshine, and low humidity, you can passively dehydrate the berries on dark blankets in the sun (remember, the berries are quick to stain, so use an old clean blanket). I have even seen a few people dehydrate elderberries by laying them out on a blanket in the bed of a pickup truck during the warm, sunny, low-humidity days of late summer!

Freezing

Freezing is another common method for preserving fresh berries. As with dehydrating, it is easier with the berries left on the umbels. You can then remove the berries with ease once frozen.

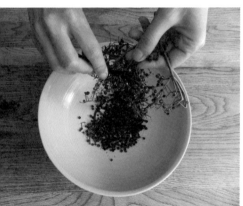

Start by rinsing your berries and spreading them on a towel to drip-dry. Place them in a clean freezer-safe collection bin or on a tray. This is a great time to remove any under-ripe or poor-quality fruit. If the bin has slats or holes, line with parchment paper or similar food-safe material. You don't want berries that fall off the stems to fall out of the bin! We generally use a dark cotton towel or old clean T-shirt. Arrange the clusters lightly in the bin.

Place the bin in the freezer as soon as possible after harvest. Allow 24 to 36 hours for the berries to fully freeze. You can wait longer, but don't go more than a week before removing the stems and placing the berries in an appropriate long-term storage bag or container.

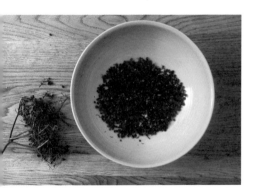

To remove the berries from the stems, wash your hands well. Pick up a cluster in your left hand and hold it inside a one-gallon freezer bag. With your right hand, remove the berries while gently shaking the cluster with your left hand. You can also use a large comb to help remove the berries. If the berries are well-frozen, they should easily fall into the bag. Being so small, they tend to thaw quickly, so it is best to remove only a small amount from the freezer at a time. This is a task best done in a cool place during the cool of the day, like early morning.

Compost the stems and any other unwanted plant material or berries. Seal the bag or container and make sure to mark the date on it. For containers, you can use a piece of tape!

Berries will keep up to 6 months in the freezer. Colder freezers, or certain styles such as chest freezers, keep the berries better than warmer freezers or upright styles. If you want to store them longer frozen, the berries will first need to be blanched, either by steam or hot water.

Juicing

Not everyone has space for a freezer full of elderberries. Another way to preserve them is by juicing. The one drawback is that the juice will begin to ferment quickly. You can refrigerate it for a week or so, freeze it, reduce it, or can it to extend the shelf life. One benefit is that juicing will reduce the amount of space elderberry takes up.

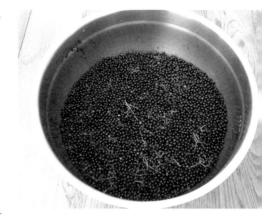

There are three ways to make elderberry juice: machine, water and heat, or steam juicing.

For the machine method start by rinsing freshly harvested berries and allow them to drip-dry on a clean towel. Prepare your juicer of choice and run the berries through, removed from any leaves, stalks, or stems. Note that many juicers and food mills struggle with elderberries—the high seed content tends to clog them up.

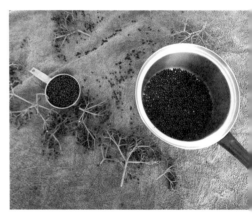

Any pulp and other leftover material make a great addition to a compost pile—don't feed raw elderberry waste to animals! Place the juice into clean or sterilized bottles and store in the refrigerator. It will keep for 7 to 10 days. Note that you shouldn't consume the juice raw.

Another method involves cooking down the fresh elderberries with additional water to produce the juice. Place your berries in a pot, adding just enough water to cover them. Bring to a boil over medium heat. Reduce to a simmer, and allow the berries to cook for 15 to 20 minutes. Remove from heat and allow to cool.

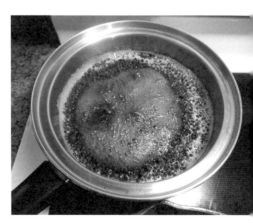

Once cool enough to handle, use a potato masher or similar tool to press the berries in the pot, breaking any remaining ones open to release their contents. Next, pour the liquid through a large strainer set over a catch pot to separate the liquid from the berries.

Now, it is time to press the berries and pulp to get every drop of goodness out of them. If needed, line the strainer with clean cheesecloth. Ladle in a few cups of berries at a time, pressing them to remove as much remaining liquid as possible. Do this until all the berries are well-pressed. We will often run the liquid through a very fine strainer one last time after pressing. You could also use a coffee filter. Bottle the juice into clean or sterilized jars and refrigerate.

Some juice recipes will include sugar or even other fruits (for additional flavor and sugar). We generally don't add any sugar, since all the ways we use the juice already involve adding sugar. If you plan to just drink the juice, adding some type of sweetener is recommended. For instance, in some Nordic countries, the juice is often made with cane sugar and apples added to the boiling water. So take this as a basic way to make juice, but feel free to experiment or adapt it to your preferences, adding various sweeteners and other fruits as desired if you don't plan to further process the juice into something else later.

A final option is to use a steam juicer—a set of pots that sit on your stovetop and use steam to extract the juice. The equipment to steam juice costs between $80 to over $200 but will save you many hours if you make elderberry creations on a consistent basis. If used properly, it also heats the berries, making the juice safe to consume straight after extraction.

To further reduce the volume and to extend its shelf life, gently simmer the juice over low heat to remove some of the water content and make a concentrated elderberry juice or pure elderberry syrup. Generally speaking, you will need to reduce the volume by half to two-thirds. This will extend the shelf life up to a month when refrigerated. When reducing the juice, take great care that it does not begin to burn on the bottom of the pan.

To extend the shelf life further, you can (carefully!) freeze the juice. One way to do so and avoid breaking bottles is to freeze the juice in ice cube trays. Once frozen, remove the cubes and transfer them to a freezer bag or storage container. If you want to make a truly shelf-stable juice, process jars by water bath canning—10 minutes for quarts and 5 minutes for pints.

Comparing the Three Preservation Methods

Dehydrating: easier than juicing, but the berries are less versatile once dried, and fairly shelf stable

Freezing: easiest, but takes the most space and has the highest ongoing storage cost

Juicing: most versatile to use, takes the least space to store, most work, further work to render shelf stable

PURCHASING ELDERBERRY PRODUCTS

If you cannot grow or forage sufficient elderberries, another option is to purchase either the berries or the juice. There are many reputable companies that now sell dried elderberries, along with syrups, juices, and other elderberry products. Fresh elderberries are much harder to come by, and outside of an occasional farmers market or roadside stand, I have rarely seen them for sale. Let's look at some words often used in association with elderberry products and what they mean.

Conventional, Wildcrafted, or Certified Organic?

People will often ask about the difference between various labels and if they matter, especially with regards to elderberry. It is a difficult question to answer. First, elderberries come from many different parts of the world. Most commercial varieties come from Europe, especially Bulgaria, though a number of other countries are also major growers. Some of them have stricter agricultural rules than the United States for what is and isn't allowed on food crops.

Conventional Berries

Conventional berries (all berries are conventional unless otherwise noted) may be grown with pesticides—this includes herbicides, insecticides, fungicides, and other chemicals. Note that many farms that grow conventional berries do not use these chemicals, or use them only on a very limited basis and as needed. But unless you are purchasing directly from the farm and the farm is honest and transparent, there is really no way to know what practices were used to tend the bushes and control weeds and pests.

Wildcrafted or Foraged

Some companies offer wildcrafted berries. Technically, such berries should come from native, unmanaged, indigenous plantings. Unfortunately, as with so-called wild blueberries, some companies unscrupulously use this designation to refer to conventionally grown berries that are from so-called wild stock.

Also note, foraged or wildcrafted berries may be exposed to significant agricultural chemicals. It just depends on their location. Wild bushes in pasture fields or woodlands are most likely very clean to pristine. Those grown along the edges of industrial row cropping or managed roadways—which are often treated with many chemicals and also expose the bushes to exhaust and other contaminants from vehicle emissions and road chemicals—are more problematic. If purchasing wildcrafted berries, I would ask the company from where and how the berries were collected and what if any rules or testing do they have in place to ensure the bushes are not exposed to the issues above.

Certified Organic

Such berries and thus their bushes must be managed in accord with current National Organic Program standards. Note that certified organic growers are allowed to use pesticides; the ones they are allowed to use come from a much shorter, restricted list. Generally, almost all chemical herbicides are not permitted under organic production, but many insecticides and other naturally derived and occurring chemicals are allowed.

If we need berries beyond what we can grow or forage, we seek to stick with certified organic. If we purchase foraged or wildcrafted berries, we ask the seller many questions about where and how they are collected. If they can't answer such questions, we find someone who can and support them with our dollars.

Preparation Methods

ELDERBERRY HAS A long history of many preparation methods, some more culinary or celebratory in nature, some more medicinal. We will cover a mixture of both.

BASIC EQUIPMENT

- Canning jars, Mason or Weck
- Mesh strainer
- Measuring cups and spoons
- Funnels
- Stock pot (useful for both water bath canning and sterilization)
- Labels: Labels are very important because without a way to mark what you made and when you made it, you may have no idea when things are ready or what they are even if they are ready!

21.* ELDERBERRY SOUP.

d.

3 pints (6 glasses) Water.
1 lb. Elderberries 4
2 ozs. (2 large tablespoonfuls) Wheat Flour . $\frac{1}{4}$
8 oz. Apples 1
4 oz. (4 tablespoonfuls) Sugar . . . . $\frac{3}{4}$
———
For 6 persons. 6

Wash the berries and boil them in 3 pints of water until they are wrinkled, strain the juice through a sieve into a basin. Then add the flour, which has been stirred with a little water into a thick paste, after which boil the apples cut up in that paste, until they are soft. Serve with rice dumplings (see No. 119) or croutons (Nos. 134, 135). Instead of the wheat flour, half the quantity of potato flour can be used ; in that case the potato flour must only be added just before serving.

▲ History is full of uses of the elderberry like this rather unique recipe for an elder soup. *WHAT TO EAT AND WHY*, 1914, ARCHIVE.ORG

404. *To pickle* ELDER BUDS.

Take elder buds when they are the bignefs of fmall walnuts, lie them in a ftrong falt and water for ten days, and then fcald them in frefh falt and water, put in a lump of alium, let them ftand in the corner end clofe cover'd up, and fcalded once a day whilft green.

You may do radifh cods or brown buds the fame way.

▲ ELIZABETH MOXON, ENGLISH HOUSEWIFERY, 1769, ARCHIVE.ORG

ELDERFLOWER FRITTERS

INGREDIENTS

6 clusters of elderberry
flowers

1 large or 2 medium eggs

½ cup beer, sparkling water,
or water

½ cup flour

Pinch of salt

Optional: powdered sugar,
cinnamon, and vanilla

Oil to fill a skillet about
½-inch deep (we prefer
palm shortening or lard)

You can substitute regular
flour with oat or another
gluten-free flour for
those wanting a gluten-
free option.

If you have an excess of flowers, or a young bush that you don't want to yet produce fruit, these are a true treat to try! Shake and pick any bugs or unwanted material off the elderflowers, but don't wash or rinse them. It washes out much of the flavor.

Directions

1. Prepare the batter by beating the eggs with the beer and salt in bowl. Add a few drops of vanilla if desired.
2. Mix the flour into the batter.
3. In a pan or cast iron skillet, warm the oil over medium heat.
4. Hold a flower cluster by the stem and dip it into the batter. Then drop the cluster into the oil, cooking until golden brown.
5. Remove from the pan and set on a paper towel for a moment to remove any excess oil.
6. Dust with sugar and cinnamon. Enjoy!

I like sprinkling cinnamon on these or adding a small bit of maple syrup or vanilla to the batter. They remind me in some ways of the funnel cakes I ate as a child at the county fair. Some people refer to these as "pancakes with handles."

Recipe adapted from: http://www.lilvienna.com/elderflower-fritters

JAMS AND JELLIES

People have consumed elderberry in jams and jellies for almost a millennium. But what is the difference between jam and jelly? Jams are made with the whole fruit, usually crushed, pulp, or purée, whereas jellies are made with fruit juice. Because elderberries contain so many seeds, jellies are the more typical preparation.

LOW-SUGAR ELDERBERRY JELLY

My friend Laurie Neverman of Common Sense Home provided these most excellent recipes and instructions for jelly. Adapted from https://commonsensehome.com/elderberry-jelly/

Directions

1. Sterilize 4 or 5 8-ounce jars; keep hot. Heat lids and rings in hot water; keep warm but not boiling.
2. Fill water bath canner and bring to a boil.
3. In a small bowl, mix together honey and pectin powder. Don't skip this step, or your pectin will clump. Set aside.
4. In a large non-reactive pot, combine elderberry juice, lime juice, and the calcium water. Bring to a full boil.
5. Add honey-pectin mixture, stir vigorously 1 to 2 minutes while cooking to dissolve pectin. Return to boil and remove from heat.
6. Ladle hot jelly into sterilized jars, leaving ¼" headspace. Wipe rims clean and screw on the lids.
7. Process for 10 minutes in water bath canner (add 1 minute for every 1,000 feet above sea level). Makes about 4 cups of jelly.

INGREDIENTS

1 quart elderberry juice
¼ cup lime juice
4 teaspoons calcium water (mixed up from a calcium powder that is included in the box of Pomona's Universal Pectin)
2 cups honey
4 teaspoons Pomona's Pectin

HOMESTYLE ELDERBERRY JELLY

INGREDIENTS

1 quart elderberry juice

4½ cups sugar

½ teaspoon butter (optional)

1 package Sure-Jell pectin

A traditional full sugar jelly made with Sure-Jell pectin.

Directions

1. Sterilize 5 or 6 8-ounce jars; keep hot. Heat lids and rings in hot water; keep warm but not boiling.

2. Fill water bath canner and bring to a boil.

3. Stir pectin into juice in saucepot. Add butter to reduce foaming.

4. Bring mixture to full rolling boil (boil that doesn't stop bubbling when stirred) on high heat, stirring constantly.

5. Stir in sugar.

6. Return to full rolling boil and boil 1 minute, stirring constantly.

7. Remove from heat.

8. Ladle into prepared jars, leaving ⅛" inch headspace. Wipe jar rims and threads. Cover with two-piece lids. Screw bands tightly.

9. Place jars on elevated rack in canner. Lower rack into canner. Water must cover jars by 1 to 2 inches. Add boiling water, if necessary. Cover; bring water to a gentle boil.

10. Process 5 minutes. Remove jars and place upright on a towel to cool completely.

11. After jars cool, check seals by pressing a finger on the middle of lids. If lids spring back, they are not sealed and refrigeration is necessary. Makes 5 or 6 8-ounce jars of jelly.

LOW-SUGAR ELDERBERRY JELLY

One final option from Laurie. Lightly sweetened with a bit of lime juice for acidity, this elderberry jelly is sure to please.

Instructions

1. Sterilize 4 or 5 8-ounce jars; keep hot. Heat lids and rings in hot water; keep warm but not boiling. Fill water bath canner and bring to boil.
2. In a small bowl, mix together honey and pectin powder. Don't skip this step, or your pectin will clump. Set aside.
3. In a large non-reactive pot, combine elderberry juice, lime juice, and the calcium water. Bring to a full boil.
4. Add honey-pectin mixture, stir vigorously 1 to 2 minutes while cooking to dissolve pectin. Return to boil and remove from heat.
5. Ladle hot jelly into sterilized jars, leaving ¼" headspace. Wipe rims clean and screw on the lids.
6. Process for 10 minutes in water bath canner (add 1 minute for every 1,000 feet above sea level). Makes about 4 cups of jelly.

INGREDIENTS

1 quart elderberry juice
¼ cup lime juice
4 teaspoons calcium water
2 cups honey
4 teaspoons Pomona's Pectin

EASY REFRIGERATOR JELLY

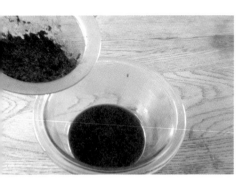

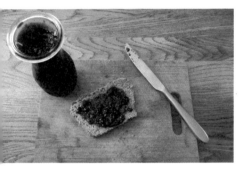

If you want to make an easy jelly that doesn't require canning and is made with honey rather than sugar, this gelatin-rich jelly is a winner.

Start by using our elderberry syrup recipe, and make the syrup without cloves, ginger, or cinnamon. Measure out one cup and place in refrigerator to chill. Next, dissolve 1½ teaspoons of gelatin into two tablespoons of the cold elderberry syrup. With the remaining cold syrup, place over low heat and gently warm while whisking in the 2 tablespoons of elderberry and gelatin. Heat the liquid to 110°F (34°C). Put into a jelly jar and place in fridge. The jelly should set in about 4 hours.

FERMENTED ELDERBERRY ENJOYMENTS

One of my favorite finds while researching this book was this almost 200-year-old book by Elizabeth Moxon.[1] It contains elder vinegar, pickled elder buds, and of course, a traditional elderberry wine.

301. To Make Elder Wine

Take twenty pounds of malaga raisins, pick and chop them, then put them into a tub with twenty quarts of water, let the water be boiled and stand till it be cold again before you put in your raisins, let them remain together ten days, stirring it twice a day, then strain the liquor very well from the raisins, through a canvas strainer or hair-sieve; add to it six quarts of elder juice, five pounds of loaf sugar, and a little juice of sloes to make it acid, just as you please; put it into a vessel, and let it stand in a pretty warm place three months, then bottle it; the vessel must not be stopp'd up till it has done working; if your raisins be very good you may leave out the sugar.

Apart from syrup or supplements, most people know elderberry because of its long history in making fermented beverages, including meads and wines. Unfortunately, I have yet to develop skills in this area of culinary craft. Fortunately, a friend of mine has such skills, and the following is a welcomed contribution from well-known mead maker and author Jereme Zimmerman.

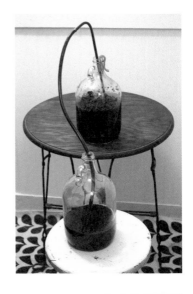

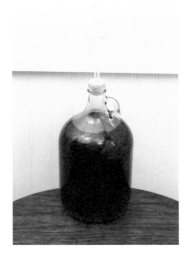

MAKING ELDERBERRY
WINE AND MEAD... LIKE A VIKING

You can make great wine or mead from pretty much any edible berry, but I like to keep at least a few bottles of elderberry in my cellar at all times. This is not only because of the excellent flavor but also because many of my wines and meads possess intentional medicinal qualities. Elderberries are chock-full of antioxidants and have antiviral and anti-inflammatory properties. As soon as cold and flu season hits, I like to head to the cellar for a bottle of elderberry mead or wine (or sometimes some peach horehound mead).

Read on and I'll help you get started making a batch of elderberry wine, mead, or both. The main difference between wine and mead is the sugar source. Otherwise, the process is pretty much the same. To produce any alcohol, you need a sugar source for yeast to feed on. A simple formula to remember is sugar + water + yeast + time = booze.

Mead is the most likely candidate for the oldest alcoholic beverage since the bees have already made the sugar source for us. All of the pollen they gathered to make the honey has yeast on it, which is dormant when honey is in its natural state, being a natural antimicrobial and preservative. Raw honey contains additional fermentation-enhancing microbes, as well as any bits of the hive that may have been left in the honey. A little bit of water makes it in, intentionally or not, and voilà! Fermentation!

For wine, most of the sugar is in the fruit (although modern wine-makers increase the alcohol content by adding sugar). Yeast is on the surface of most fruits, waiting to eat any sugars it can get its greedy little... (mouths?) on, but the fruit is ahead of the game with its thick protective skin. As soon as it starts to rot, though, the skin softens and yeast can begin to make its way in. Monkeys and other animals are known to travel for miles following the smell of rotted fruit, not only because they know it will provide them with needed nutrients but also because chowing down on semi-boozy fruit makes them feel quite nice. Making wine is simply a process of controlling and speeding up this process.

Beer is also an ancient beverage; archeologists are beginning to discover that it was being made much earlier than they had originally thought. It is made primarily from grains, and grains have a much tougher exterior covering the starches inside produced by germination. Moisture and heat while grains are at the peak of germination, and a bit of grinding of the grains, is needed to turn the starches into sugars and produce alcohol. Hence, most of the earliest alcohols were a hybrid of mead, wine, and beer. People knew that if you mixed enough sugars together in some water and helped it ferment, they would produce a nutritious, soul-enlivening beverage. Over time we developed names and styles for these beverages, one of the oldest being the Latin *biber*, a generic term for "drink," which eventually morphed into "beer."

Equipment

To make any kind of alcoholic beverage, you'll need some equipment. While beer requires some specialized equipment, wine and mead have less specialized needs. For sure, there is lots that you can invest in, but we'll be talking about 1-gallon batches, which can be made using the following basic kitchen equipment:

- 1 2-to-3-gallon cooking pot and stir spoon
- 1 2-to-3-gallon open-mouthed container or 1-quart jar (optional; only required for wild fermentation)
- 1 or 2 1-gallon glass jugs (you can get by with one, but an extra is handy for when you need to transfer your mead or wine to a new vessel)
- 1 airlock (cheap plastic device that can be purchased from a home-brew store) or balloon (accomplishes the same thing as the cheap plastic device)
- Funnels of varying sizes with a screen, filter, cheesecloth, or colander
- Food-grade vinyl tubing for siphoning

Ingredients

I'll provide you with a list of ingredients for a basic 1-gallon batch of mead or wine. You can modify these a bit and even add herbs, other fruits, etc., for future batches. For both of these, you will produce a product that verges between semi-sweet and dry. The alcohol level should reach around 10 to 12 percent ABV (alcohol by volume). You can increase the sweet or dry factor by adjusting the sugar/honey levels, but keep in mind that less will result in a slightly lower alcohol content. You can add as much as 1 pound more of sugar or honey, but I don't recommend adding that until the *secondary fermentation* phase (see below), as you'll essentially be dropping a bunch of kids in a candy store, resulting in overstressed yeast that will produce off flavors or stop fermenting altogether.

Process

The process is almost exactly the same for wine and mead. When selecting yeast, you have a wide range of options. All commercial yeast started out wild. Historically, people would start by drawing in wild yeast from the air and on the skins of fruit and other botanicals they were fermenting. Over time, they would breed stronger yeasts that would impart a certain flavor profile and alcohol level by reusing the yeast from a previous batch, or drying it and passing it down as a family heirloom. Nowadays, we have people in white coats to isolate single strains in a laboratory that consistently produce certain flavors and alcohol levels. The sheer variety of yeast options out there can be overwhelming, but they'll pretty much all do the job. Most mead makers use wine yeast, so for both mead and wine, if you purchase yeast, look for yeast that will produce your desired flavor profile (some are better for sweeter meads/wines and others for more on the dry end). A good one to start with for both mead and wine is Lalvin D-47 (semi-sweet), although I sometimes use Lalvin EC-1118 (dry/champagne) or Lalvin ICV - K1-V1116 (good for sparkling fruit wines/meads). Bread yeast will also do the job, although it can't always reach levels of above 10 percent ABV, and some feel it imparts too much of a yeasty flavor. Beer and ale yeast will work as well, but you'll need to lower the sugar content to produce something more akin to a gluten-free beer or cider.

If you choose to use wild yeast, I cover working with it in detail in my books *Make Mead like a Viking* and *Brew Beer like a Yeti*, but the process on its own is quite simple. A rare few have reported to me that their wild yeast experiments don't produce much more than 6 to 7 percent ABV, but for the most part, working with wild yeast is just a matter of using enough sugars to reach the desired alcohol content.

You can combine all of the ingredients for a full batch (minus yeast) in a 2- to 3-gallon wide-mouthed container or create a yeast starter in a pint or quart jar to use with multiple batches. Essentially, what you'll be doing is stirring at least a couple of times a day and covering the vessel with a cheesecloth or dish towel. This provides aeration, which is essential for the yeast to get to work. Once you've got an active ferment in 3 to 5 days (you'll know when you stir and get some fizz and a bit of foaminess), you can switch to an airlocked container. The yeast are now alive and happy and can thrive in an anaerobic (without air) environment as opposed to the aerobic (with air) environment in an open container. That's the process in a nutshell. My website (www.jereme-zimmerman.com) has a trouble-shooting guide in the blog section titled *Wild Yeast Is Your Friend*.

Instructions

Whatever yeast you choose to work with, follow these steps for making your elderberry wine or mead:

1. Gather your ingredients and clean your equipment. Modern mead and wine makers stress heavy sanitation of all equipment the mead or wine will touch, but I simply clean and rinse well with hot water as I would with cooking. I do sometimes use an environmentally safe cleanser called One Step No Rinse Cleanser.

2. Bring a little under 1 gallon of water to a simmer and then cut off the heat. For wine, stir in all sugar now and be sure to stir to keep it from sticking to the bottom and caramelizing. For mead, wait about 15

minutes, as you don't want to kill off beneficial yeast and microbes; also, too much heat will dissipate some of the aroma in the final product. For both mead and wine, what you have now is officially *must*.

3. Squeeze and drop in the half lemon or other citrus and add all other ingredients.

4. Allow the must to cool (covered) to room temperature (60° to 70°F [15° to 21°C]). A couple of hours or overnight should do.

5. If wild fermenting the entire batch, follow the procedure for aerating the must in an open-mouthed container to draw in wild yeast.

6. Next, pour everything but the lemon through a funnel into a glass jug, leaving 4 to 5 inches headspace. You want a lot of aeration at this point, so swirl the jug after you pour.

7. Add desired yeast directly to the must.

8. Place an airlock or balloon on the jug opening. This allows the CO_2 that is produced through the fermentation process to escape (preventing explosions or severe gushing!), but keeps outside air from entering and depositing acetobacter, acetic acid bacteria that will produce vinegar over time. You have now started the *primary fermentation* phase.

9. In 3 to 4 weeks, you'll want to *rack* (from a French wine-making term for "transferring between vessels") off the solid ingredients into another jug. This begins the *secondary fermentation* phase. For fruit wines and meads, I usually add a bit more fruit (about 1 cup per gallon), as much of the fruit flavor will have dissipated during vigorous primary fermentation. Although I've never had a problem, for elderberries, it's best to heat them in water first, as they contain trace elements of a toxic glucoside cyanide compound that can be removed by heating. Fill the vessel with additional water if needed to about 1 inch below the opening. Don't use chlorinated tap water, as the chlorine will kill the yeast.

10. You'll need to rack once more in about 2 months if you want a clarified wine or mead. Gathered on the bottom will be a yeast cake, also known as *lees*. Each time you rack, place your siphoning tube just a

bit above the lees to leave them behind. They can be tossed in the compost, used to start a new batch (some of the yeast will still be alive), or even made into a salad dressing.

11. Throughout this period, keep the jug in a dark, warm area (around 60° to 70° F [15° to 21°C]). Between 4 to 6 months (when you see no further CO_2 activity), do a final racking into a vessel with a spigot and prepare to bottle.

12. You can use various bottles. If you've invested in a corker, use wine bottles and corks (fill the bottle to leave about ¾" below the cork), or if you have a capper, use non-screw-top beer bottles. Or, use swing-top bottles or wine bottles with screw-on lids (don't reuse beer screw-top bottles; they're too flimsy and unreliable). For the latter options, fill to about ½" below the opening.

Now is when you get to exercise your patience! Although some mead and wine can taste good at bottling, it all improves with age. Try to give it at least 4 to 6 months, or sneak a bottle to sample early to see how the flavor improves over time. Regardless of when you drink it, be sure to share with friends and belt out your preferred toast. Mine is of course the Viking/Scandinavian *skål!*

▲ *THE CHEMIST AND DRUGGIST*, 1930, ARCHIVE.ORG

ELDERBERRY KOMBUCHA

Many years ago, kombucha became one of our family's favorite home-fermented drinks. The base drink—fermented sweet tea—marries well with a wide variety of additional flavors provided by herbs, spices, and so many other inputs and options. One variety we especially like involves elderberry.

Instructions

1. Take 13 ounces of fresh unflavored kombucha (preferably homemade, but you can try this with store-bought as well).
2. Add 2 ounces of elderberry juice or pure elderberry syrup (not the medicinal kind that contains honey!).
3. Add ½ teaspoon grated ginger.
4. Pour into a stoppered bottle and allow to sit in a dark, warm place (72° to 75°F [22° to 24°C]) for 2 to 3 days.

Enjoy! After about 3 days, the mixture should become nicely fizzy. If it hasn't, it means the bottle either wasn't tightly sealed or wasn't in a warm enough location.

OTHER WAYS TO PREPARE ELDERBERRY

People have enjoyed elderberry in both alcohol-based fermented beverages and regular ones for thousands of years. Both have their place and their own unique benefits. The main difference between a tea and syrup is the strength of the solution and the amount of sweetener.

"Yes, I believe you have," said his mother. "If one drinks two full cups of hot elder tea, one usually gets into the warm countries!" Then she tucked the bedclothes carefully around him so that he wouldn't take cold. "You've had a nice nap while I was arguing with him as to whether that was a story or a fairy tale."

"And where is the Elder Tree Mother?" asked the boy.

"She's in the teapot," said the mother. "And there she can remain!"

Hans Christian Andersen "The Little Elder-Tree Mother"

Elderberry flowers and berries both make great additions to teas. The main difference is that flowers, which don't have the stomach-upsetting issues of the berries, can be gently steeped rather than needing to simmer. Both have a long history of use in teas.

Instructions

1. Place ½ tablespoon of dried elderberries in 2 cups of water with some rose hips or any other desired herbs or flowers.
2. Bring to a gentle simmer for about 10 minutes. Strain out and compost plant materials or feed to appropriate animals.
3. Enjoy as is or with a dab of honey or other added sweetener.

ELDERBERRY FOR ANIMALS?
People aren't the only ones who appreciate elder! As far back as it was used for people, it was also used for livestock. However, raw elderberry shouldn't be given to your livestock. While some wild animals do well on the raw berries, there are warnings about giving them to domesticated animals. At the same time, the leftovers from making elderberry juice, syrup, and many other creations are an amazing addition to your poultry, pig, or pasture-raised animals' diets. They will improve the color and flavor of their meat and fat, while also improving their overall health. Moderation is key: for chickens, about 1 ounce of elderberry pulp per chicken per day; about 1 pound for pigs and other animals. Any remaining beneficial material in the pulp, they will happily make use of and, in exchange, turn it into fertilizer and fantastic meat and eggs. If you don't have animals, it is also an excellent addition to your compost or worm compost.

INGREDIENTS

1 dozen large elderflower
    cymes (clusters of
    flowers)

2 cups honey (you can also
    use solid sugars like
    sucanat or white)

1 lemon, sliced

1 ounce citric or tartaric
    acid, optional

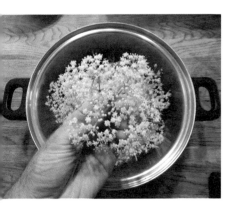

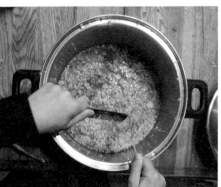

Another way to make use of flowers the first few years a new bush is getting established, elderflower cordial has hundreds of years of history.

Instructions

1. Pick clean clusters of elderflowers. Remove as much of the stalks/stem as possible.
2. Submerge the flowers in the water. Add the lemon slices to the water. You can also add some lemon zest (grated rind) if desired. Allow to sit for 12 to 24 hours.
3. Strain the mixture, pressing as needed to extract as much juice as possible. Pour the liquid into clean bottles.
4. Store in a refrigerator for up to 2 weeks or freeze.

This makes a lovely base for many other creations; for instance, by adding some water and optional gelatin, you can make elderflower popsicles or sorbet. Or you can boil various fruits—such as apricots, peaches, or plums—in the cordial to make a sauce.

Adapted from *Nature's Playground* by Fiona Danks and Jo Schofield, Chicago Review Press, 2007.

ELDERBERRY-INFUSED HONEY

Herbal honeys have a long history. What could be better than taking an amazing honey and marrying it to many wonderful herbs and spices, both preserving the herbs and creating a delicious addition to your condiment collection?

It is very important with herbal honeys to use sterile, dry containers—moisture can cause spoilage, fermentation, or other problems.

INGREDIENTS

⅓ cup Amercian elderberries

⅔ cup honey

Ceylon cinnamon stick, optional

Instructions

1. Place herbs into the bottom of a pint jar.
2. Pour honey over the herbs. Note that the herbs will absorb some of the honey, so you may need to add more honey to the jar. For this reason, use a jar that is slightly larger than the amount you are making, so you have space to add honey.
3. Allow to sit for 2 to 4 weeks in a warm, dark place. It is best to occasionally flip the jar or stir it. Depending on the type of jar, it's a good idea to place it on a plate in case some honey leaks.
4. After it has sat a few weeks, place the jar in warm (approximately 105° to 110°F [40.5° to 43°C]) water for 10 to 20 minutes. This will soften the honey so that you can then strain out the berries or other herbs. Once strained, rejar and enjoy!

You may be wondering what to do with the leftover herbs. One option is to use them to make tea! Since they will already contain a fair bit of honey, I would do it on low heat and note that you shouldn't need to add any sweetener.

ELDERFLOWER WATER AND SYRUP

The first two years, you may opt to collect the flowers from newly planted bushes instead of letting them go to fruit. What do you do with the flowers? Make elderflower water and syrup, of course!

The process for both is quite simple.

Process

Begin by bringing 8 cups of water to a simmer. Add 4 cups of elderflowers. Allow to simmer for about 20 to 30 minutes—the water will turn a marvelous golden color. Reduce the liquid by about half, down to 4 cups.

For elderflower water, strain the liquid and pour into bottles. It will keep refrigerated for about a week.

For syrup, after straining the liquid, return it to the pot. Over low heat, add 1 cup of sugar or other sweetener and whisk thoroughly. The longer you heat it, the thicker the syrup. It will last 3 to 4 weeks in the refrigerator.

ELDERBERRY SYRUP

Most people in America meet elderberry for the first time as a suggested way to treat colds and flu, especially in the winter. What makes it into a syrup is the sweetener—generally ½ viscous sweetener by volume, sometimes less, sometimes more. Traditionally, honey was the most common option, but we also enjoy using maple syrup and date syrup. If you plan to give children under the age of one any, then only use an alternative sweetener because of the botulism risk that honey poses to their immature digestive systems. Alternative sweeteners are also important for those on certain diets. You can even make a less sweet version by decreasing the amount of sweetener—it will just result in a thinner, more watery final product.

INGREDIENTS
(USING FRESH BERRIES)
1 cup fresh elderberries
1½ cups clean water
½ cup real honey
Optional: 2 Ceylon
    cinnamon sticks or ½
    tsp Ceylon cinnamon:
    5 cloves: ginger, ½
    inch fresh grated or ¼
    teaspoon dried

Instructions

1. Bring 1⅓ cups of water to a simmer.
2. Add all the ingredients except honey.
3. Cover and allow to simmer for 30 to 60 minutes.
4. Strain mixture through a fine sieve or colander, pressing the excess liquid out of the berries and other ingredients. The leftovers are great for chickens, pigs, worms, or the compost pile!
5. Measure the amount of liquid; you should end up with about 1 cup. If needed, add some water to get to 1 cup; this helps speed cooling process.
6. Allow the strained mixture to cool to 110°F (43°C).
7. Add sweetener of choice and blend mixture with a fork or small whisk. If the sweetener is especially thick, you may need to use a handheld blender on a low setting to thoroughly incorporate it. Makes 16 ounces or 1 pint.

Low-Honey/Sweetener Version

For medical or other reasons, some people need or want to restrict their sugar/carbohydrate intake. In such a situation, use ⅓ to ½ less sweetener and make a thinner, but still delicious, syrup. Note that the

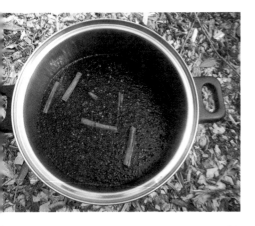

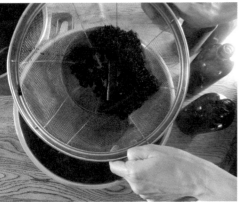

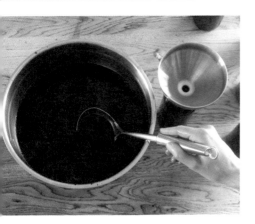

total final volume will be less, or you will need to make slightly more liquid to add the sweetener to reach a full pint.

Other Syrup Versions

If using dried berries, follow the recipe above, but use ½ cup of dried berries in place of fresh. Makes one pint.

If using regular elderberry juice, use 1 cup of juice + ⅓ cup water and only simmer for approximately 15 to 20 minutes with the additional ingredients.

For concentrated juice or syrup, use ½ cup juice and a bit over ¾ cup water.

Feel free to consult commercial product labels as well, as products will vary.

Syrup Storage and Shelf Life

Elderberry syrup is best stored in a cool, dark place, preferably the refrigerator. Since the sweetener is not pasteurized in our recipe, the risk of fermentation or mold is greater than with pasteurized products, both store-bought or homemade.

The syrup should last at least 4 to 6 weeks, though we and many others have had it last 8 to 12 weeks in the coldest part of the fridge.

If you want to make a larger batch, say from your own fresh berries, and save it for winter use, you can freeze the syrup. I would suggest freezing it in no more than 1-cup portions, enough to last a few days when thawed, in a square Pyrex dish or an ice cube tray. Store frozen portions in a freezer bag or larger container.

Alternative Sweeteners

While honey is usually the sweetener of choice for syrups, many other options are available. Maple syrup, date syrup, and the like all make wonderful elderberry syrup, with some added benefits. For instance, children under the age of one shouldn't consume raw honey, so an elderberry syrup made with an alternative sweetener is infant friendly, unlike the honey version. Some people, because of dietary beliefs, such as vegans or vegetarians, may want to avoid honey. Others can consume date or other sugars, but not honey or maple syrup.

If you substitute into an alternative sweetener, here are a few guidelines.

- Few sweeteners are as sweet as honey. It is almost twice as sweet as most other common sweeteners, like maple syrup, so the final product will have a similar amount of total carbs/sugar but may taste less sweet.
- The final thickness/viscosity will vary based on the sweetener. In our experience, maple syrup makes a thinner final product, whereas date syrup makes a thicker one. The thicker the sweetner, the thicker the syrup; the thinner the sweetener, the thinner the syrup.
- Sweetener costs vary substantially, both between sweeteners and depending on your location. You may want to adjust the amount in the recipe based on cost considerations. In our area, honey is almost half the cost of maple syrup, but in other places, the reverse may be true.

Other Possible Ingredients

With most recipes in this book, you should treat them as more like suggestions or guidelines. For instance, the above is a basic elderberry recipe. Many other ingredients are possible: rose hips for extra vitamin C, echinacea, and more! So don't feel constrained by the suggested recipes.

Extending the Shelf Life: A Little Bit of Brandy Makes the Elderberry Go Down

Since the honey in traditional syrups isn't heated, over time the mixture will start to ferment. Fermentation is a tricky thing, and can produce amazing results or all sorts of problems. Before refrigeration, people relied on a very old solution—the addition of alcohol—to inhibit fermentation.

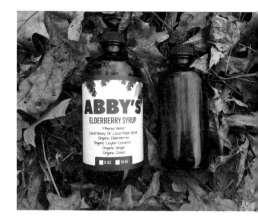

▲ Dark, amber glass bottles are the best way to store syrups and similar herbal preparations.

THE EVERY-DAY COOK-BOOK.   239

ELDERBERRY SYRUP.

Take elderberries perfectly ripe, wash and strain them, put a pint of molasses to a pint of the juice, boil it twenty minutes, stirring constantly, when cold add to each quart a pint of French brandy; bottle and cork it tight. It is an excellent remedy for a cough.

▲ Before refrigeration, other tools, such as alcohol, were used to keep foods from spoiling. *THE EVERY-DAY COOK-BOOK*, 1889, ARCHIVE.ORG

Historically, rather large amounts of alcohol were sometimes added—like in the cookbook pictured above, where the final syrup would contain ⅓ alcohol by volume. If the original alcohol used was 80 to 120 proof (40 to 60 percent ABV), the final syrup would be 12 to 20 percent ABV alcohol.

This much isn't necessary to extend the shelf life; at about 10 percent, you get a substantial increase. This would mean for 1 quart of syrup you add 1 cup of alcohol—you want something that is around 80 proof (40 percent), so that the final product will end up around 20 proof (10 percent) alcohol.

If you do use alcohol, make sure that you stir the mixture well to ensure that it thoroughly combines; the syrup, liquid, and alcohol will naturally want to separate, but a good mixing will help bind it into a nice even solution. For those who don't want to use alcohol, especially if giving large doses to small kids, another option to extend shelf life is to add a small amount (⅓ to ½ cup to 1 quart syrup) real apple cider vinegar. Some people and kids may find the vinegar adversely affects the flavor, others may not.

TINCTURES

A tincture is either an alcohol- or glycerin-based method of extracting various chemicals from plant materials. In the case of glycerin, heat is usually also employed. Some plant compounds are extracted by both methods, but some compounds are better extracted by one over the other. For those who for personal or religious reasons cannot or won't consume alcohol, or for small kids, glycerin tinctures are a great option. An added appeal is their sweet taste, which makes them especially appealing to children.

Alcohol tinctures are generally quite easy to make. Their main drawback is time—generally 1 to 6 months is suggested or needed to create a quality tincture. For elderberry tincture, stick with an alcohol that is 80 to 120 proof (40 to 60 percent). We prefer a certified organic alcohol, either vodka or rum.

ALCOHOL ELDERBERRY TINCTURE

We just finished up a batch of elderberry tincture, and I have to admit, I see why elderberry and alcohol go together—he flavor is most refreshing, especially if you are using a good-quality alcohol for the extraction. Here is how we did it.

INGREDIENTS

2 cups of dried elderberries

750 mL of organic alcohol

Directions

1. Clean a 1-quart glass jar, thoroughly rinse, and dry. Place alcohol and elderberries in the jar.
2. Shake well. Place in a cool, dark location, such as a closet or pantry.
3. Once or twice per week, shake mixture well.
4. Allow to age for 2 to 6 months.
5. Once the mixture is mature, strain and bottle. It is best to store tinctures in dark amber bottles in a cool, dark place. Light may damage and degrade many of the beneficial compounds floating around in the alcohol.

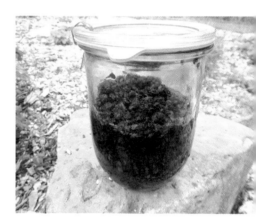

We prefer putting the tincture into dropper bottles. Unlike syrups and other preparations, where you consume a few tablespoons at a time and many ounces per day, alcohol tinctures are generally consumed a few drops at a time. Dropper bottles make it easier to get small amounts without loss and put a few drops into small mouths as well.

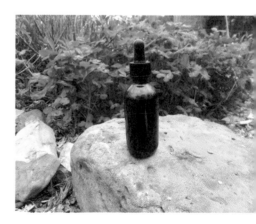

Saving on Organic Alcohol

Alcohol is expensive. One way to save is to purchase higher-proof organic alcohol in bulk—a gallon or more. It is generally available as 180 proof, or 90 percent, alcohol. You will then need to "thin" the alcohol back to 80 to 120 proof, 40 to 60 percent, for tincture making. By our estimates, this cuts the cost of the alcohol in half or more compared to buying small bottles from stores.

To get back to the proof or percent alcohol you need requires some high-quality distilled water and some basic math.

If you are not too particular, the easiest way is to combine them half and half (so 2 cups distilled water and 2 cups alcohol) to make a 45 percent proof alcohol. For a slightly lower proof, start with just a few spoonfuls less than 2 cups alcohol and add a few spoonfuls extra water, and you will end up around 40 percent. Generally speaking, almost all good tinctures are made with at least 40 percent, 80 proof or higher, alcohols.

To make a 120 proof, 60 percent alcohol, you will need to use ⅔ cup of alcohol for each ⅓ cup of distilled water. If you want to get really precise, break out pencil, paper, and your algebra! Note, all these numbers depend on the starting proof of the alcohol you are using. If it is higher or lower than 180, mathematical adjustments will be needed! Generally, it is best to err on the side of a slightly higher alcohol content.

Although glycerin tinctures are more work than alcohol-based ones, they take a great deal less time to get a final product—a few days instead of a few months. The speed is achieved by using very low heat over the course of many hours or days to hasten the extraction.

Glycerin is made from fat, generally vegetable fat such as coconut, soy, palm, or others. Whether to pay extra for certified organic depends on which fat the product is made from—if soy, rape (canola), or other modern industrial crops, definitely go organic. Stick with pharmaceutical grade if possible, but at the least, ensure that what you purchase is food-grade. Pharmaceutical grade is guaranteed with regards to greater purity, in terms of heavy metals, other contaminants, and microorganisms. An added bonus, vegetable glycerin is currently far less expensive than alcohol, especially organic alcohol.

If you have a crock-pot with a low setting or, even better, one that you can set to a specific temperature, in our experience it is the safest and easiest way to make glycerin tinctures. While you can do it on a stovetop, letting things cook overnight was a risk we were not willing to take.

Directions

1. Prepare your jars. Make sure they are well dried.
2. Place berries and other ingredients in the jars. Cover the mixture with glycerin. Seal the jars with their lids.
3. Place the jars in the crock-pot. Fill the crock-pot with water, leaving the top inch or so of the jars uncovered—you don't want the water sitting over their tops. You also don't want the water sitting below the level of the mixture in the jars.
4. Some will place an old clean washcloth on the bottom of the crock-pot to protect the jars from possibly cracking from close contact to the heating elements. This is a prudent step, especially for older crock-pot models that do not allow easy temperature regulation.

INGREDIENTS
2 cups food- or pharmaceutical-grade glycerin
1 cup elderberries
Optional: Ceylon cinnamon stick

EQUIPMENT
Crock-pot, ideally one with good temperature control
1 quart or 2 1-pint Mason jars, washed and well rinsed

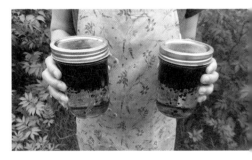

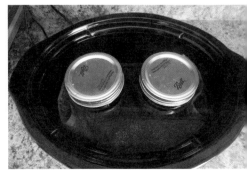

5. Leave the jars in the crock-pot for 2 to 3 days. Add more water to the crock-pot as needed.
6. Once finished, remove the jars from the crock-pot. Allow the jars to cool for 30 or more minutes before handling.
7. Strain out mixture and rebottle.
8. Store tincture in a cool, dark place out of direct sunlight.

For tinctures, dark amber dropper bottle jars, available in 1- to 4-ounce sizes, are generally the preferred method of storage. Unlike syrups, which are taken in moderate quantities of a few spoonfuls per day, tinctures are generally consumed at much lower doses.

A Note on Sterilization

You can improve the shelf life or reduce the risk of spoilage of all syrups, tinctures, and other such products by sterilizing the jars or containers. This is usually done by boiling the jars for at least 10 minutes. If you live at higher altitudes, for each 1,000 feet above sea level, add 1 minute. If you have a pressure canner or Instant Pot, you can also use those to sterilize your tools and containers.

Just note that sterilization only works if your entire work area is clean—if you remove the jars and set them on surfaces or touch with hands, tools, towels, or anything else that isn't also sterile or clean, you immediately reintroduce all sorts of microorganisms. Thus, sterilization is no substitute for creating a clean work area and practicing good hygiene when handling or making edibles or medicinals. I especially suggest using a "segregated" preparation rule. We do not do personal cooking or other such tasks while making medicinals or large batches of preserved products. We set aside time and kitchen space, we thoroughly clean the entire kitchen and work areas, and we only use the kitchen and work areas for the preparation of the particular things we have scheduled. This helps stop all sorts of mistakes and other possible problems, and generally allows the entire process to go much faster and far more successfully than otherwise.

For making syrups and tinctures, we use a high-quality natural soap and warm water, along with a great deal of care in creating a clean work area when making such medicinal things. Some people may prefer or some situations may call or require you to employ full sterilization. Just remember, sterilization cannot replace cleanliness and good habits!

Preferred Jars for Tinctures

We love the Weck all-glass canning jars for fermenting, canning, and tincture making. The all-glass body and lid with simple stainless steel metal sealing clips are hard to beat. The only non-glass/metal component is the sealing ring. In our experience, Ball Mason jars have a few drawbacks. First, they sometimes leak or seep, especially when shaken, and they cannot be turned and left upside down. Given how labor-intensive and ingredient-expensive these preparations are, loss isn't something that we want to allow, nor the mess that loss creates.

Second, they easily succumb to rust and other forms of failure. A few too many times, we have opened a Mason jar to find the top rusting into the contents below. With Weck or similar jars, you will never have this issue. Last, the chemicals used in the lids of Ball jars are cause for some concern. The metal lids are coated with BPA or BPA-free chemicals, but studies have found that these BPA-free lids may actually contain more and more dangerous chemicals than the standard, already problematic, BPA ones.

One way to alleviate the rust and other concerns is to use the Mason jars with Tattler-style lids instead of the standard metal ones that Ball and other companies sell and provide. The Tattler lids are suitable also for canning, and are durable and reusable.

ELDERBERRY HAM AND BBQ GLAZE

GLAZE INGREDIENTS

¾ cup of sucanat or
      brown sugar
2 tablespoons elderberry
      juice, syrup, or jelly
¼ cup brown mustard
1 tablespoon cider vinegar
Cloves

Either as a stand-alone glaze or an addition to other sauces and marinades, this is another excellent use for elderberry juice or jelly. For a stand-alone, take 1 tablespoon of a sugar-free elderberry juice and add 1 teaspoon of maple syrup or honey. Mix thoroughly, add any other spices, a bit of mustard, or whatever else you desire, and use it as a glaze on chicken or pork. Elderberry also goes well with duck.

Instructions

1. Preheat oven to 350°F (177°C).
2. Start with a five to eight pound smoked, cured ham. Score the top of the ham in diamonds, placing whole cloves in each diamond into the ham. Place ham on platter or baking rack, and put into oven for an hour and a half.
3. Meanwhile, mix together 1 cup of elderberry jelly, ¼ cup of brown mustard, and 2 tablespoons of apple cider vinegar. If using the refrigerator jelly, you can add an additional two tablespoons of brown sugar. Pour mixture on the scored part of the ham, and bake an additional 30–45 minutes. Every 10 minutes, using a spoon or baster, remove liquid from the baking dish to baste ham.
4. Remove from oven, allow to cool for 15 minutes before slicing. Strain liquid in baking dish, or pour as is over the ham slices or into a dish to serve as a sauce to go along with the meal.

Note: if you use a jelly instead of a juice or syrup, you may need to reduce the amount of sweetener. Take the above as suggestions, not rules, and adjust to your preferences.

If you have elderberry jam, it can be spread on many types of meat alone or mixed with mustard, spices, and other ingredients while the meat is baking to add flavor or create a glaze.

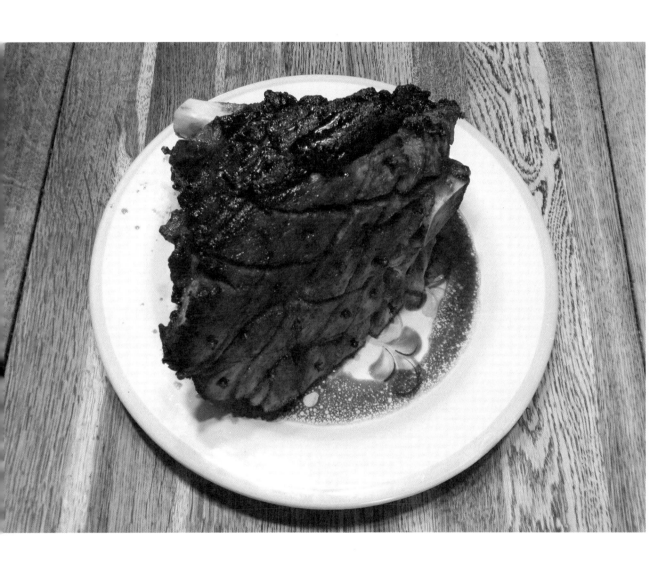

ELDERBERRY CREAM CHEESE FROSTING

This particular recipe creates a pale pink frosting with a light elderberry flavor. This works best with American elderberries if you want a bright, pinkish color. European produce a darker, purple-brown tint.

Instructions

1. Start by making elderberry juice by boiling ½ cup of water with 1 quarter cup dried (1 cup fresh) elderberries. Boil for approximately 10–15 minutes. Press and strain mixture. Then, return to heat and reduce until only ¼ cup of liquid remains.

2. In a food processor, cream 8 ounces of cream cheese with ¼ cup of white sugar. Add more sugar if you desire a sweeter frosting. Next, add 1¾ cup of heavy cream. Process until mixture thickens, but don't over process as it will cause the ingredients to separate. Next, stir in 3 to 4 tablespoons of the elderberry mixture. You can now either use it immediately or chill the mixture in the fridge.

OTHER USES FOR ELDERBERRY PULP

A few of my friends will use the pulp leftover from making syrup to create flavored beverages for cooking, as a holiday pick-me-up, and more.

For instance, you can take the pulp and cover it with red wine. Allow it to sit for a few weeks, then strain out the wine, and press the pulp (to remove the excess liquid that the pulp will have absorbed), and chill. the drink is good both cold and warmed up.

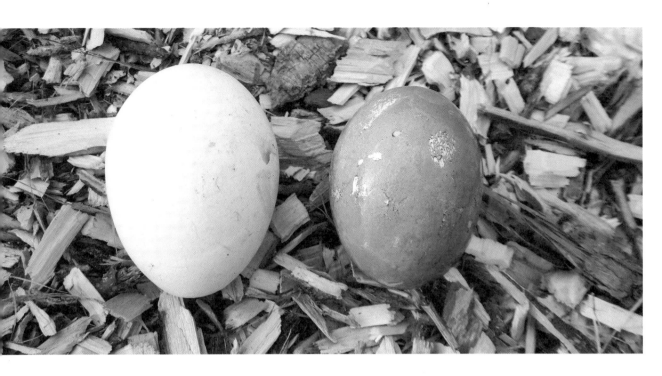

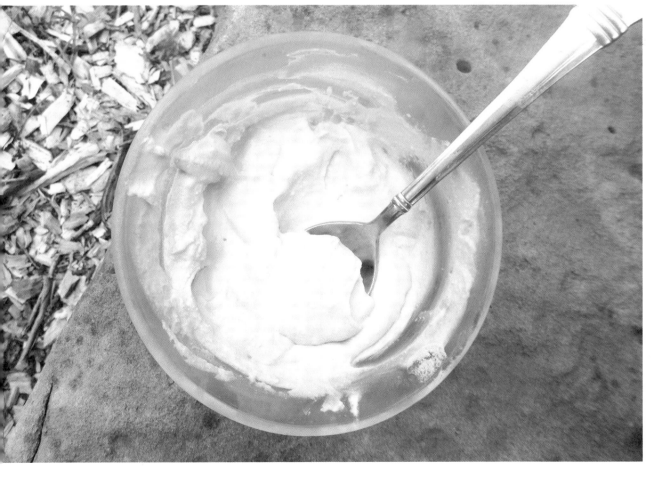

Crafts and Other Uses for Elder Wood

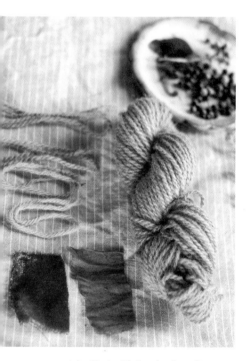

ELDERBERRY IS MUCH more than a food or medicine. The potent chemicals found in the plant serve many other purposes, such as in dyes or natural insect repellants. The wood of the elder historically was used in everything from furniture and flutes to amazingly fun children's toys. This is just a brief look at some of the crafts and ways you can create from elder. Dozens more are possible, from pipes to gimlets, from little storage jars to small figurines and toys.

Pruning an elder results in a large amount of waste wood. What should you do with it? At the very least, compost. But why not instead turn it into additional useful things to enrich your life and the lives of others?

CHILDREN, CYANIDE, AND ELDERBERRY CRAFTS

As mentioned earlier, elder is a toxic plant. It contains many potent chemicals, some that form cyanide as they break down. These chemicals are present in all parts of the plant: roots, bark, wood, leaf, and berry. Because of this, some people warn against allowing children to have elder crafts that they put in their mouth, such as whistles, flutes, and similar creations. Others find this concern overstated as, historically, children across many parts of the world would have used many elder toys and wood instruments, with no reported issues. Personally, I think this warning is without merit, unless you have a child

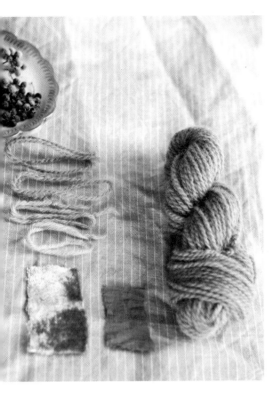

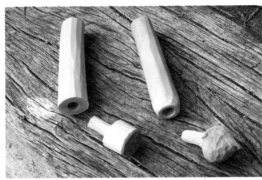

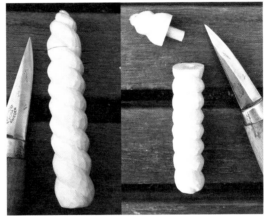

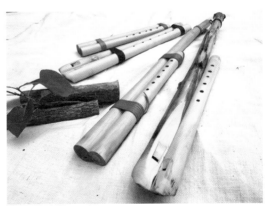

▲ A single elder branch can create multiple long pieces of wood, each suitable for different crafts. This one branch will become a popgun, a few whistles, and more. JULIA BILLINGS, WWW.WOOLENFLOWER.COM

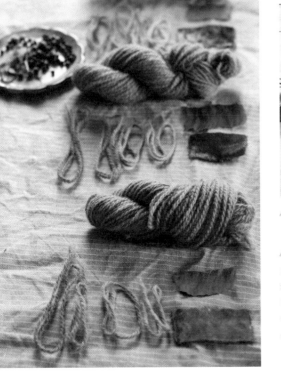

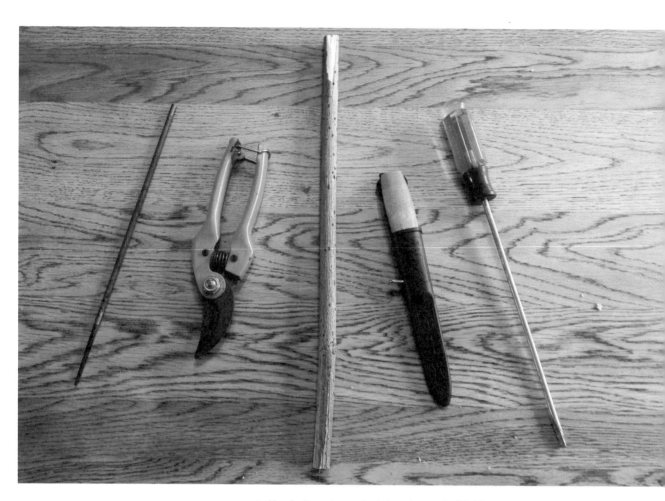

▲ You don't need many tools to make wonderful elder creations.

that will chew heavily on something made of elder. So, for very small children, especially when teething or if they have a bad habit of biting or chewing on things, elder may be of concern. For everyone else, I say elder away!

Also note: traditionally, crafts were made from dried or dead rather than fresh green wood. Many Native American and European techniques involved drying fresh wood before using in crafts if that was their starting material. My hunch is this helps reduce any risks associated with the wood, and it also helps ensure your creations don't crack or break because of drying, but it is not something we have any research on currently.

WHAT YOU WILL NEED

You need a limited number of tools—a good carving or whittling knife, a few different sizes and lengths of screwdrivers, and a round file—these are especially useful for removing the pith! Longer, smaller screwdrivers are the best, and you can often find used ones for just a dollar or so at yard sales, thrift stores, and pawn shops. Some sandpaper or sanding sponges in various grits is needed.

A hacksaw is also exceptionally useful for cutting down longer branches to desired lengths; in our experience, when you try to use plant shears, it causes the hollow elder branches to crack along their length. For longer creations, it is unlikely you will find a sufficiently long screwdriver to remove the pith. In such situations, you can use heavy-gauge wire or, one of my favorites, an old practice-tipped arrow that has lost its fletching. These are often about 30 inches in length, allowing you to clean out 3- or 4-foot pieces of elder. A power drill is also useful for starting holes or certain cuts into the wood, such as for making whistles or flutes. Realize your crafting with elder will improve with time, so if your first few attempts don't turn out well, don't be discouraged!

If you have additional tools, like a Dremel, don't hesitate to use them when and where appropriate. But don't let access to only a few tools stop you from making use of your elder wood.

ELDER WHISTLE

Whistles are one of the oldest uses of hollow woods in human history. If people didn't use elder, they used bamboo or one of dozens of other species. Also, they let you make use of pieces of elder wood that are too crooked or twisted for longer creations. To make a whistle, you will need a piece of wood about 3 inches long. Thoroughly remove the pith—you want the stem to be "as clean as a whistle." You should also remove the bark with either a knife or, my preference, sandpaper or a sanding sponge which is safer and more efficient, especially for kids.

Once you have a piece of the right size and length, about ¾ inch (2 cm) from one end, you need to notch out the whistle hole. Do this

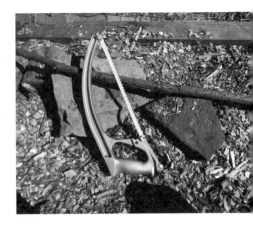

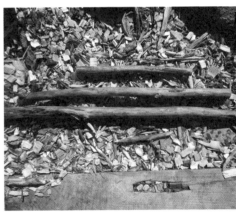

▲ A single elder branch will provide numerous pieces of wood, each suitable for different projects and purposes.

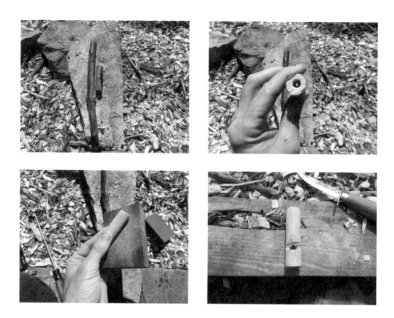

by first making a vertical cut on the side closer to the end and then a horizontal cut. You may need to sand after making the cuts to create a nice clean hole.

The whistle won't sound nice (yet!). You need to make a dowel to fit into the mouth end that goes from the end right to the edge of the hole. Look for a branch just slightly larger than the end hole, remove the bark and shape it down until it snugly fits. Once you have a good fit, on the top side of the dowel, shave it flat by removing just a small amount of the wood. This flat side faces up in the flute, directing air toward the hole. You may need to try a few times by inserting, testing, then removing and trimming down the dowel until you are happy with the sound. Remember, you can always remove more, but you can't add it back once you trim it off!

Make another dowel to serve as a stopper on the other end of the whistle, again going for snug fit. Once you are happy with the sound and the dowels, give it all a good sanding. Then, finish it with your choice of food-grade oil.

ELDERBERRY FLUTE

As a young child, I remember learning to play a plastic recorder in grade school. You can make something far more beautiful using some of the pruned elderberry wood. Elder flutes are found across history, and in many parts of Europe are still made and used. The flutes made from elder wood go by many names and come in many styles—the *koncovka* in Slovakia, a *sampogna* in Italy, and *corworas* in some Native American dialects, to name just a few.

The scientific name for elderberry, *sambu*, is the Latin word for "flute," a tribute to one of the plant's earliest non-edible uses.

WHAT YOU WILL NEED

1 dry piece of elder, about ¾ to 1¼ inches in diameter and 14 inches long

Knife

Flat-head screwdriver

Drill or similar tool to make holes (a hand drill or power drill)

Round file or small-diameter screwdriver

Instructions

1. Start with some dry, relatively straight pieces of elder wood. Using a hacksaw or similar tool, cut it to about 14 inches.
2. Use a round file and screwdriver to remove the inner pith from the wood.
3. The hole spacing depends on the person using the flute. The general recommendation is to start by finding the middle of the flute and place your thumb there. Using your other hand, place your four fingers, two on either side of your thumb, along the wood. Use a pencil to mark those spots. They should be about one thumb-print width apart.
4. Now, use the tool of your choice to create the four finger holes, with your pencil marks as a guide. You can either leave or remove the bark. If you remove the bark and want the flute to last, apply some sort of finish. Make sure you use food-grade, food-safe materials to finish. I prefer tung oil and citrus solvent, as it tends to bring out the natural beauty of any wood.[1]

ELDERBERRY BELLOWS

Elderberry's association with fire is also quite ancient. Some think that *aeld* was used for elderberry since the hollowed stems make an excellent bellows. Because we heat with wood, fire making is an

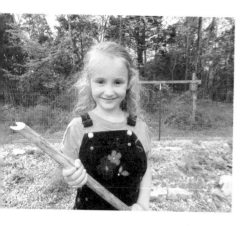

almost daily occurrence 3 to 5 months of the year. Sometimes, you just need to get a bit more air to start a new fire or get a bed of coals back going. An elderberry bellows is a great and simple tool to have on hand to help with the task. This is really just a long flute without the holes, so there is no need to give detailed instructions. You want a much longer final product—in the 24-to-36-inch range—to keep yourself well back from the fire.

ELDER LANCE OR SPEAR

As a child, I grew up on a street that dead-ended into the Mill Creek Park system. In a 5-minute run, we found ourselves surrounded by lakes, creeks, streams, waterfalls, rock formations, and woods, even though we were in the midst of the city. Fishing, hunting crawdads and salamanders, and so much else filled our summer days. The late 1800s was quite similar, when *The American Boy's Handy Book* gave kids plans for an elder lance to help them catch small animals and fish instead of having to use their hands!

Start with a fairly straight piece of elder that is approximately 2 ½ to 3 feet long, longer or shorter depending on the size of the child. Cut the smaller end at a steep angle of around 60 degrees, like a quill point. Old books used a two-prong tip to the lance, which you create by cutting a V shape on the lower side of the pointed tip.

You can remove the bark and sand and finish the spear, or just keep it as is, an annual toy renewed each spring after the old one was broken or otherwise lost or discarded during adventures and play. If you have access to very long and straight pieces of elder wood, you can even make spears suitable for spearfishing and hunting small animals by adding barbs or a true tip to the end.

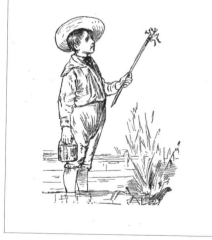

▲ For everything from vampires to frogs, the elder lance is a tool with a long and rich history. *THE AMERICAN BOY'S HANDY BOOK, 1862*

ELDERBERRY PENCILS

Another fun craft is making old-style pencils out of elderberry wood. Note that, generally, these are more decorative than practical in nature. This is a fun use for smaller-diameter elder wood.

Instructions

By now you know the drill. Cut the elder down to length and remove the pith. Then fill with either the charcoal or craft pencil fill. Pencil lead comes in many sizes, so you may want to measure a few hollowed out pieces before ordering so you get a nice snug fit. Once filled, use your whittling knife to sharpen the pencil tip like a typical pencil. My children found this craft especially fun, and the pencils, while not practical for everyday use, make a fun gift or decoration.

BLOWGUN/POPGUN

While probably not the first use for elderberry, a blowgun is likely one of the earliest. Everyone from Pliny to Culpeper mentioned young children's proclivity to use elder wood to make a toy for shooting objects at other kids!

I can remember me and other kids using straws to shoot things at my siblings or other unsuspecting children. I can imagine children from early America and Europe shooting all sorts of objects out of hollowed elderberry branches.

Elder makes both a good blowgun and popgun. What is the difference? A blowgun is powered by you blowing air into it. A popgun is powered by using a "ram" to drive one object in the barrel toward another object, creating air pressure that quickly builds and then, "pop," causes one of the objects to fly out of the barrel. Hence its most fitting name.

Like most elder creations, both start the same, find an appropriate segment of wood, 8 to 12 inches. It doesn't need to be perfectly

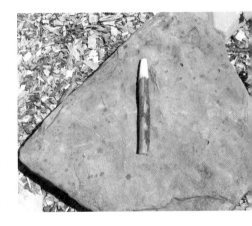

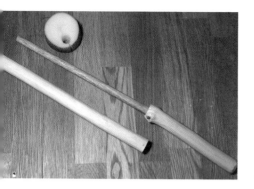

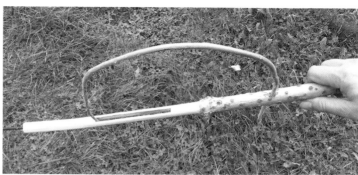

straight, but the straighter the better it will perform. Remove the pith. For a blowgun, at this point, you are done.

For a popgun, you now need to either find or make the ram, a long round rod. This was traditionally made from a whittled piece of a different wood. Unless you are experienced, this can take a bit of time. Another option is to find an old screwdriver or similar tool or very large piece of heavy-gauge metal wire (like off a cattle or hog panel). With a screwdriver, you may need to beat the tip round; a flat head and many other shapes, instead of serving as a ram, will skewer whatever you put into the barrel.

To operate the popgun, use two small wads of paper or two pieces of potato or apple will work. Load both ends of the barrel. Just use it like a cookie cutter on a piece of potato or apple you have cut into about ¼ inch slices. Once both ends are loaded, on the side you plan to run the ram, push the piece slightly farther in with the ram. Then, ready, aim, ram! Push the ram quickly through the wood, and you should find yourself enjoying a millennium-old use for elder. As you drive the ram forward, pressure builds between the two pieces, until, "pop," and one projectile flies forth.

How to Make Elder-Guns.   203

a quill as a nozzle to my "squirt" it would throw water much further than the others. It is a very simple thing to make a good squirt-gun, and one may be manufactured in a few minutes.

First cut a joint from a piece of an old cane fishing-pole, being careful not to disturb the pithy substance that almost closes the hollow at the joints. Insert a quill for a nozzle at one of the joints and see that it fits tightly; leave the other end open. With your pocket-knife fashion from a piece of pine or cedar the plunger (B, Fig. 132); leave the wood a little thicker at both ends and wrap a rag around one end, making it just thick enough to fit snugly in the cane after wetting it. This completes the "squirt" (A, Fig. 132). To use it, immerse the quill in water, first push the plunger in, then draw it out slowly until the gun is filled with water. Take aim, and when you push the plunger back again the water will issue from the quill in a sudden stream, travelling quite a distance. One of these water-guns is quite useful in the garden; by its means the insects infesting the rose bushes and other shrubs may be knocked off in no time. When the owner of an aquarium finds dead animals or plants that should be removed, located in some crack or cranny that is difficult to reach, the squirt-gun is just the thing to dislodge the objects without disturbing the surrounding rocks or plants.

FIG. 132.—Cane Squirt-Gun.

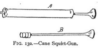

FIG. 133.—A Simple Elder-Gun.

Elder-Guns and Pistols.

When the author was a very small boy he was taught by some playmates to make an elder gun, a simple contrivance, made of a piece of elder or any other hollow stick. A long

Notes

Chapter 1: History

1. Hippocrates of Cos. *Affections*. https://www.loebclassics.com/ view/hippocrates_cos-internal_affections/1988/pb_LCL473.193. xml?rskey=sXR8r6&result=1&mainRsKey=IDmzVV

2. Hippocrates of Cos. *Diseases*, Vol. 2, https://www.loebclassics. com/view/hippocrates_cos-diseases_ii/1988/pb_LCL472.201. xml?rskey=dKy4iu&result=1&mainRsKey=KarI3P

3. Hippocrates of Cos. *Affections*.

4. Nicholas Everett. *Alphabet of Galen: Pharmacy from Antiquity to the Middle Ages*. University of Toronto Press, 2012, P. 229.

5. Theophrastus. *Enquiry into Plants*. https://www.loebclassics.com/ view/LCL079/1916/volume.xml, pp. 200–201.

6. Dioscorides. *De Materia Medica*, Vol. 4, pp. 729–730, http://www. cancerlynx.com/BOOKFOURROOTS.PDF

7. Pling the Elder. *On the Materials of Medicine*, http://www.perseus. tufts.edu/hopper/text?doc=Perseus%3Atext%3A1999.02.0137%3A-book%3D24%3Achapter%3D35

8. http://www.perseus.tufts.edu/hopper/text?doc=Perseus%3Atex-t%3A1999.02.0137%3Abook%3D15%3Achapter%3D7

9. M. Baker. *Discovering the Folklore of Plants*, Buckinghamshire, UK: Shire Publications, 1928, pp. 52–56.

10. W. Milliken and S. Bridgewater. *Flora Celtica: Plants and People in Scotland*. Edinburgh: Birlinn, 2004.

11. Maud Grieve. *A Modern Herbal: The Medicinal, Culinary, Cosmetic and Economic Properties, Cultivation and Folk-lore of Herbs, Grasses, Fungi, Shrubs, & Trees with All Their Modern Scientific Uses*, Vol.1. Courier Corporation, 1971, p. 269.

12. Michael Ettmeuller. https://books.google.com.

13. Edward Hamilton. *The Flora Homoeopathica: Or Illustrations & Descriptions of the Medicinal Plants Used in Homoeopathic Remedies*, 1852, p. 455, accessed from https://books.google.com/books

14. Hans Christian Anderson. "The Little Elder-Tree Mother," 1895, http://www.andersen.sdu.dk/vaerk/hersholt/TheElderTreeMother_e.html

15. Lady Rosalind Northcote. *The Book of Herbs*, 1903, https://archive.org/details/bookofherbs00nort/page/184

16. Nicholas *Culpeper's. The Complete Herbal*, 1850.

17. http://www.gutenberg.org/files/49513/49513-h/49513-h.htm

18. K. Pejml, 1938. Cited in I. Salamon and D. Grulova: https://www.researchgate.net/profile/Ivan_Salamon/publication/308026477

19. Lydia Maria Child. *The American Frugal Housewife: Dedicated to Those Who Are Not Ashamed of Economy.* University of Leeds Library, 1835.

20. Dr. Thomas Faulkner and Dr. John H. Carmichael, *The Cottage Physician.* https://archive.org/details/cottagephysician92faul/page/4

21. Ibid., p. 146.

22. Elizabeth Moxon. *English Housewifery: Exemplified in above Four Hundred and Fifty Receipts Giving Directions for Most Parts of Cookery*, 1741.

23. C. Hart Merriam. *The Dawn of the World*, http://www.sacred-texts.com/nam/ca/dow/dow14.htm

24. J.N.B. Hewitt. *A Constitutional League of Peace in the Stone Age of America: The League of the Iroquois and Its Constitution*, 1920, p. 539.

25. *The Herb Society of America's Essential Guide to Elderberry.* http://www.herbsociety.org/file_download/inline/a54e481a-e368-4414-af68-2e3d42bc0bec

26. Joseph Jacobs. *Some of the Drug Conditions during the War between the States, 1861–1865*, 1898.

27. Bacchus and Emilie Lebour-Fawssett. *New Guide for the Hotel, Bar, Restaurant, Butler, and Chef: Being a Handbook for the Management of Hotel and American Bars, and the Manufacture of the Principal New and Fashionable Drinks*. London, UK: W. Nicholson and Sons, 1884.

29. Ortha L. Wilner, "Roman Beauty Culture," *The Classical Journal*, Vol. 27, No. 1 (Oct. 1931), pp. 26–38.

30. John Worlidge. *Systematic Agriculture: The Mystery of Husbandry Discovered*, https://archive.org/details/acompleatsystem00worlgoog/page/n5, pp. 149/195.

31. *Some of the Drug Conditions during the war Between the States, 1861–1865*. A paper read before a meeting of the American Pharmaceutical Association held in Baltimore, MD, in August 1898, by Joseph Jacobs, Pharmacist, Atlanta, GA.

Chapter 2: Description, Anatomy, Terminology, and Nutrition

1. Samuel Thayer. *Nature's Garden: A Guide to Identifying, Harvesting, and Preparing Edible Wild Plants*. Bruce, WI: Foragers Harvest Press, 2010, p. 399.

2. https://www.ncbi.nlm.nih.gov/pmc/articles/PMC5372600/; https://kundoc.com/pdf-advanced-research-on-the-antioxidant-and-health-benefit-of-elderberry-sambucus-n.html; https://www.ncbi.nlm.nih.gov/pmc/articles/PMC3056848/#B; http://www.ncbi.nlm.nih.gov/pmc/articles/PMC4848651/; http://omicron-pharma.com/pdfs/ElderberryClinicalOJPK_Published.pdf; http://www.ncbi.nlm.nih.gov/pubmed/15080016

3. http://uncommonfruit.cias.wisc.edu/american-elderberry/

4. https://hort.purdue.edu/newcrop/ncnu07/pdfs/charlebois284-292.pdf

Chapter 3: Cultivation and Care

1. https://www.ncbi.nlm.nih.gov/pmc/articles/PMC4863952/

2. https://midwest-elderberry.coop/overview/charlebois_elderberry-botan.pdf, 12.

3. https://www.nrcs.usda.gov/Internet/FSE_PLANTMATERIALS/publications/mipmcrj11674.pdf

4. http://uncommonfruit.cias.wisc.edu/american-elderberry/

5. https://catalog.extension.oregonstate.edu/em9113; http://www.northeastipm.org/about-us/publications/ipm-insights/how-to-trap-spotted-wing-drosophila/; http://www.midwest-elderberry.coop/cultivation/vinegar-to-trap-swd.pdf; http://www.midwest-elderberry.coop/cultivation/pests--problems.html

6. http://www.missouribotanicalgarden.org/gardens-gardening/your-garden/help-for-the-home-gardener/advice-tips-resources/pests-and-problems/insects/mites/eriophyid-mites.aspx

Chapter 4: Harvesting, Foraging, and Preserving

1. USDA Forest Service. http://www.fs.fed.us/wildflowers/plant-of-the-week/cicuta_maculata.shtml.

Chapter 5: Preparation Methods

1. Elizabeth Moxon. *English Housewifery: Exemplified in above Four Hundred and Fifty Receipts Giving Directions for Most Parts of Cookery*, 1741.

Chapter 6: Crafts and Other Uses for Elder Wood

1. https://exotic-instruments.wonderhowto.com/how-to/craft-native-american-flute-out-elderberry-360325/; http://www.howcast.com/videos/334239-How-To-Make-a-Native-American-Flute; http://urbanorganica.typepad.com/urban_organica/2009/02/making-elderberry-flutes.html

Additional Reading and Resources

HAVING COMBED OVER and consulted dozens of works and hundreds of articles and texts, some modern and many ancient, for this book, I commend a few in particular for your further enjoyment.

First, the Herb Society of America has an excellent publication all about elderberry, *The Herb Society of America's Essential Guide to Elderberry*. You can find it on their website, www.herbsociety.org

Second, Denis Charlebois has what is considered the best resource for those hoping to grow elderberry at a commercial scale, *Elderberry: Botany, Horticulture, Potential*. It is available free at the Midwest Elderberry Cooperative website, another excellent resource about commercial elderberry production. https://midwest-elderberry. coop/overview/charlebois_elderberry-botan.pdf

Unfortunately, a great deal of historical elderberry research and writing in Europe is in languages I cannot yet read and are not available currently in English. So while I could peruse and enjoy Latin, Greek, and other historical works from Europe that are available in English, I had to rely on secondary resources to explore this area of elder lore. One of the best essays I found on this subject is "Elderberry (*Sambucus nigra*): From Natural Medicine in Ancient Times to Protection against Witches in the Middle Ages: Brief Historical Overview," I. Salamon and D. Grulova by, Department of Ecology,

Faculty of Humanities and Natural Sciences, University of Presov, Presov Slovak Republic, 2015.

For those interested in foraging, Samuel Thayer and Arthur Haines each have excellent books that include discussions of elder. Thayer has three books on the subject and Arthur two.

About the Author

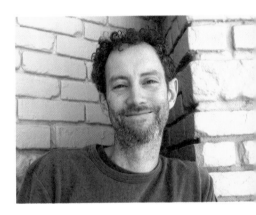

JOHN MOODY IS the founder of Whole Life Services and Whole Life Buying Club. He is the director of Steader and previously served as the executive director of the Farm-to-Consumer Legal Defense Fund. Involved with farming, food, and homesteading over the last decade, including running an elderberry syrup business, John is a well-known speaker at numerous conferences and events, such as Mother Earth News and Wise Traditions. He won the 2013 Weston A. Price Activist of the Year award and is one of two old-timers and five rambunctious kids who farm and homestead on 35 acres in Kentucky.

A NOTE ABOUT THE PUBLISHER

New Society Publishers is an activist, solutions-oriented publisher focused on publishing books for a world of change. Our books offer tips, tools, and insights from leading experts in sustainable building, homesteading, climate change, environment, conscientious commerce, renewable energy, and more—positive solutions for troubled times.

We're proud to hold to the highest environmental and social standards of any publisher in North America. This is why some of our books might cost a little more. We think it's worth it!

- We print all our books in North America, never overseas
- All our books are printed on **100% post-consumer recycled paper,** processed chlorine free, with low-VOC vegetable-based inks (since 2002)
- Our corporate structure is an innovative employee shareholder agreement, so we're one-third employee-owned (since 2015)
- We're carbon-neutral (since 2006)
- We're certified as a B Corporation (since 2016)

At New Society Publishers, we care deeply about *what* we publish—but also about *how* we do business.

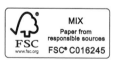

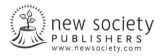

www.newsociety.com

New Society Publishers
ENVIRONMENTAL BENEFITS STATEMENT
For every 5,000 books printed, New Society saves the following resources:[1]

19	Trees
1,752	Pounds of Solid Waste
1,927	Gallons of Water
2,514	Kilowatt Hours of Electricity
3,184	Pounds of Greenhouse Gases
14	Pounds of HAPs, VOCs, and AOX Combined
5	Cubic Yards of Landfill Space

[1]Environmental benefits are calculated based on research done by the Environmental Defense Fund and other members of the Paper Task Force who study the environmental impacts of the paper industry.